Sewerage and Sewa
Environmental Health Issue

This book examines the increasingly prevalent issues around sewerage and sewage and explores what environmental health practitioners (EHPs) can contribute to addressing this issue and what further action is required.

The book sets out an analysis of the contents of raw sewage, including what should not be flushed away, explaining that householders who flush non-flushable products into the sewerage system contribute to the problem (and also give the water and sewerage companies an excuse). The work explains the terminology used and will also examine the legal issues that have arisen from failure of the UK sewerage system to operate or be operated as intended to protect public health. The operation of the privatised water and sewerage companies in England and Wales and the regulatory system to which they are supposedly subject is scrutinised along with an examination of what EHOs/ EHPs can do to address the problems that lead to sewage from homes and businesses polluting the environment. The book considers what has been called regulatory failure, what reforms and investments are needed, and what EHPs can do to bring pressure on other agencies and policy makers to ensure that untreated sewage does not end up polluting to environment.

This book is essential reading for all environmental health practitioners, but also anyone keen to learn more about the issues surrounding the increasingly volatile UK sewage system and the companies and institution involved in its operation and governance.

Stephen Battersby, MBE, is an environmental health practitioner, independent consultant, and advisor.

Routledge Focus on Environmental Health
Series Editor: Stephen Battersby, MBE PhD, FCIEH, FRSPH

Assessing Public Health Needs in a Lower Middle Income Country
Sarah Ruel-Bergeron, Jimi Patel, Riksum Kazi and Charlotte Burch

Fire Safety in Residential Property
A Practical Approach for Environmental Health
Richard Lord

COVID-19: The Global Environmental Health Experience
Chris Day

Regulating the Privately Rented Housing Sector
Evidence into Practice
Edited by Jill Stewart and Russell Moffatt

Dampness in Dwellings
Causes and Effects
David Ormandy, Véronique Ezratty and Stephen Battersby

Tackling Environmental Health Inequalities in a South African City?
Rediscovering Regulation, Local Government and its Environmental Health
Practitioners
Rob Couch

Leadership Lessons from a Global Health Crisis
From the Pandemic to the Climate Emergency
Jo Nurse

Sewerage and Sewage as an Environmental Health Issue
Stephen Battersby

Sewerage and Sewage as an Environmental Health Issue

Stephen Battersby

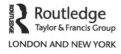

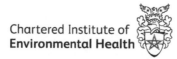

LONDON AND NEW YORK

First published 2024
by Routledge
4 Park Square, Milton Park, Abingdon, Oxon OX14 4RN

and by Routledge
605 Third Avenue, New York, NY 10158

Routledge is an imprint of the Taylor & Francis Group, an informa business

British Library Cataloguing-in-Publication Data
A catalogue record for this book is available from the British Library

ISBN: 978-1-032-44619-6 (hbk)
ISBN: 978-1-032-45157-2 (pbk)
ISBN: 978-1-003-37564-7 (ebk)

DOI: 10.1201/9781003375647

Typeset in Times New Roman
by codeMantra

Contents

Table of cases

Series preface

This is the fourteenth publication in the series, with more in the pipeline. This edition reflects an issue, some aspects of which have hit the headlines. How we deal with sewage has always been an environmental health issue and indeed local government has its origins in attempts to improve public health by protecting water sources from contamination by human waste. These days, waste contains many pollutants in addition to microorganisms that can affect health, but this volume questions whether we have the infrastructure and investment that will protect environmental and public health.

The aim of the series remains as ever; to explore environmental health topics, traditional or new, and raise sometimes contentious issues in more detail than might be found in the usual environmental health texts. It is a means by which environmental health issues can be discussed with a wider audience in mind.

This series is an important part of the professional landscape, as is apparent from the titles published so far. Environmental health practitioners (EHPs) bring their expertise to a range of situations and are deployed differently, but not always to the best effect so far, as public health is concerned. All too often, politicians, both at the national and local levels, are unaware of what environmental health is, what practitioners do, or how they work. It is common that practitioners have a 'low profile' or are taken for granted. It is hoped that this series will be used as a means of highlighting the work of EHPs.

We want to encourage readers and practitioners, particularly those who might not have had work published previously, to submit proposals, as we hope to be responsive to the needs of environmental and public health practitioners. I am particularly keen that this series is seen as an opportunity for first-time authors, and as ever, I would urge students (whether at the first- or second-degree level) to consider this an avenue for publishing findings from their research. Why, for example, should the hard work that has gone into a dissertation or thesis lie unread on a library shelf? We can provide advice on turning a thesis into a book. Equally, this series can be a way of extending a presentation, paper, or training material, so that it can reach a wider audience.

The series provides a route for practitioners to improve the profile of the profession as well as provide a source of information. It has the advantage of having a relatively quick turnaround from submission of the manuscript to publication and can be more up to date and immediate than a standard textbook or reference work.

It seems that EHPs have perhaps not been good at telling others about their work. To be considered a genuine profession and to develop professionally, EHPs on the front lines need to "get published", writing up their work of protecting public health. This series is a route for analysing actions and reporting on what worked in practice, what was successful, what wasn't, and why. This can provide useful insights for others working in the field and also highlight policy issues of relevance to environmental health.

Contributing to this series should not be seen merely as an exercise in gathering Continuing Professional Development (CPD) hours but as a useful method of reflection and an aid to career development, something that anyone who considers themselves a professional should do. I am pleased to be working with Routledge to provide this opportunity for practitioners.

As has been made clear it is not intended that this series takes a wholly "technical" approach but provides an opportunity to consider areas of practice in a different way, for example, looking at the social and political aspects of environmental health in addition to a more discursive approach in specialist areas.

Our hope remains that this is a dynamic series, providing a forum for new ideas and debate on environmental health topics. If readers have any ideas for titles in the series, please do not be afraid to submit them to me as series editor via the e-mail addresses below.

"Environmental health" can be taken to mean different things in different countries around the World, and so we welcome suggestions from a range of professions doing "environmental health" work or policy development. EHPs may be a key part of the public health workforce wherever they practise, but there are also many other practitioners working to safeguard public and environmental health. It is hoped that this series will enable a wider range of practitioners and others with a professional interest to access information and also to write about issues relevant to them.

Forthcoming monographs are likely to cover such topics as the effectiveness of housing regulation, air pollution, and monitoring private water supplies. We are in contact with colleagues around the world, encouraging them to submit proposals. That does not mean we have no need for further suggestions; quite the contrary, so I hope readers with ideas for a monograph will get in touch via Ed.Needle@tandf.co.uk.

Stephen Battersby MBE PhD, FCIEH, FRSPH
Series Editor

Introduction

In the UK and most of Europe, we rely on a water carriage system for our sewerage system to work.[1] The amount of sewage will therefore be a reflection of water use, which has increased significantly over time. For example, the amount of water used by the average household in the UK has increased by 70% since 1985. Almost 50% of the UK's water is used in the homes.[2] Recent figures show how water usage is increasing; in 2016, this was 139 litres; in 2021, the average household used 152 litres per day.[3] At the same time, it has to be remembered that much of the infrastructure that carries this waste from our homes would have been installed at least 50 years ago. According to the English Housing Survey[4] 72% of England's dwellings were built before 1980. When it leaves our homes, sewage becomes the responsibility of the water and sewerage companies(WaSCs); whether they have met their responsibilities or been made to do so is something that will be considered. Yet it is a matter of out of sight out of mind until something goes wrong, and as in the case of storm water overflows, pollution becomes apparent.

One aim of privatisation was to increase investment in the water and sewerage infrastructure. As the paper published in 2023 notes [1], the level of investment in the sewerage system has been inadequate and certainly insufficient to meet public health and environmental demands.

How the WaSCs discharge their responsibilities (or don't) is what has been hitting the headlines. In England, WaSCs discharged raw sewage into the rivers of England and Wales from combined sewer outfalls that are monitored (and not all are) more than 400,000 times in 2020, according to the Environment Agency. Although this improved in 2022 to over 300,000, drier weather was a major factor, not investment by the companies, and this still represents massive pollution of our waters.[5] Untreated effluent, including human waste, wet wipes, and condoms, was released into waterways for nearly two million hours in 2022. Such discharges pose a risk to public health and the ecosystem. As the 2022 Report from the House of Commons Environmental Audit Committee [2] said a "chemical cocktail of sewage, agricultural waste [beyond the scope of this work], and plastic is polluting the waters of many of the country's rivers" and "water companies appear to be dumping untreated or partially treated sewage in rivers on a regular basis" so "cleaning up our rivers is important for public health and vital to protect wildlife".

In July 2021, Southern Water was fined a record £90 million for deliberately dumping billions of litres of raw sewage into protected seas over several years for its own financial gain. This was headline news, and again during the summer of 2022, sewage pollution of beaches and coastal waters as the result of sewage outfalls made the headlines[6] and various newspapers started campaigns.

Surfers Against Sewage, who have been campaigning to end sewage for over 30 years, reported that 9,216 sewage discharge notifications were issued between October 2021 and September 2022, and sewage was discharged into designated bathing water over 5,000 times during the 2022 bathing season (15 May–30 September).[7] This is clearly a major environmental health issue.

Over the summer of 2022, Ministers published a strategy outlining how they would tackle what they call the "unacceptable" levels of sewage discharge. This is discussed in Chapter 5. An investigation by *The Telegraph* newspaper earlier in 2022 found that water companies are releasing raw sewage into rivers more than 1,000 times a day, despite this supposedly limited to when there is heavy rainfall.

The quality of our environment and particularly recreational waters is a public and environmental health issue, but sewage (rather than agricultural run-off) starts its journey into these waters much closer to home and is generated by us all. This is where local authority EHPs have a traditional role. There may be other circumstances where EHPs can contribute to addressing this problem, which risks the UK regaining its epithet as the "dirty old man of Europe". These are also addressed in this book.

It remains a function of EHPs to help prevent the escape of sewage into the environment (including the ground) from drainage, where it poses both a risk to public health and the ecosystem. While this book does not claim to be a legal text, it is inevitable that there is much reference to Cases, not least because that is the basis for determining the status of a pipeline carrying sewage and also whether or not a problem can be dealt with by EHPs and local authorities.

Notes

1 According to the European Environment Agency households account for about 10% of total water consumption in the whole of the EU. The figure may be significantly higher in urban areas and areas with poor water resources. On the basis of information from four countries, about one third of this is for personal hygiene, one third for washing clothes and dishwashing, 25 to 30% for flushing toilets and only about 5% for drinking and cooking.

2 https://www.internetgeography.net/topics/how-has-the-demand-for-water-in-the-uk-changed/ and it should be noted that in 1950 only 46 per cent of households had bathrooms which indicates that water consumption was much less,

https://www.theguardian.com/society/2018/mar/21/british-homes-without-bathroom-archive-1950

3   https://www.statista.com/statistics/1211708/liters-per-day-per-person-water-usage-united-kingdom-uk/

4   https://www.gov.uk/government/statistics/english-housing-survey-2021-to-2022-headline-report/english-housing-survey-2021-to-2022-headline-report

5   https://www.gov.uk/government/news/environment-agency-publishes-event-duration-monitoring-data-for-2022andhttps://environment.data.gov.uk/dataset/21e15f12-0df8-4bfc-b763-45226c16a8ac

6   See, for example, https://www.bbc.co.uk/news/science-environment-62574105

7   https://www.sas.org.uk/water-quality/water-quality-facts-and-figures/

References

1   Giakoumis T and Voulvoulis N, 2023, Combined sewer overflows: relating event duration monitoring data to wastewater systems' capacity in England, *Environmental Science: Water Research & Technology*, Advance Article. DOI: 10.1039/D2EW00637E

2   House of Commons Environmental Audit Committee, 2022, Fourth Report of Session 2021–22 "Water Quality in Rivers", HC74.

1 Sewage, sewerage, definitions, terms, and important agencies

Sewage and its contents

The pipelines, the infrastructure, whether drains or sewers, are known as sewerage. The contents of foul sewers and drains are "sewage" (see definitions below). As Dr Rob Collins of the Rivers Trust said in evidence to the House of Commons Environmental Audit Committee [1], discharges from combined sewer overflows (CSOs) "combine raw sewage with what runs off the urban environment", potentially comprising "a huge chemical cocktail: faecal microbes (bacteria and viruses), hydrocarbons, industrial chemicals, plastics, pharmaceuticals, and personal care products" with unknown effects on human health if swallowed. The plastics include microplastics, and the viruses include polio. This will be discussed in more detail in Chapter 2, which looks at the public and environmental health implications of sewage discharges.

While it may be seen as semantics to distinguish between a sewer, a drain, and sewage, and the general public might use the terms interchangeably, EHPs ought to have a better understanding of the terms as this will be an important consideration when investigating a problem and so is dealt with first in the next section.

Definitions, terminology, etc.

A drain or a sewer? What is the difference, and does it really matter?

This definition is out of alphabetical order because it is of fundamental importance. As this book will spell out, the ultimate responsibility for the condition (and contents) will largely depend on this distinction.

The history of public health legislation shows how the terms sewer and drain begin to be used more precisely, but not always helpfully. The 19th-century sanitary legislation is the true starting point. The Public Health Act of 1848 used the word 'drain', to identify a passage for the outflow of sewage from a single building. The term 'sewer' meant any system of drainage that

DOI: 10.1201/9781003375647-1

was not a 'drain' though both could contain sewage and/or surface water. The Public Health Act of 1875 refined the definitions. Although that Act is not operative, the definitions contained within it may remain relevant in cases today, as it can still be necessary to refer to them in order to establish the current status of specific conduits. The adage "once a sewer, always a sewer" holds true, as we shall see.

To the layperson, the difference between a drain and a sewer may seem a matter of semantics, but it does have implications for legal responsibilities, and indeed, it has not been unknown for water and wastewater companies (WaSCs) to attempt to avoid their responsibility by arguing that a pipeline was a drain, not a sewer. On the very first page of Garner [2], quoting Mr Justice Wills from a case heard in 1896 and referring to "sanitary legislation", it was considered "futile" to "extract from the various details of the legislation a set of harmonious principles always underlying the specific provisions". It is not much better, almost 130 years later.

It has generally been regarded that a sewer is a pipe that serves more than one premises, whereas a drain serves only one premises or building. Section 219(1) of the WIA'91 provides that "'drain' means ... a drain used for the drainage of one building or of any buildings or yards appurtenant to buildings within the same curtilage". Any other pipeline would be a sewer. Yet the Court of Appeal has held that a pipe constructed as a sewer remained a sewer and not a drain even though it received effluent from only one property (*Bromley LBC v Morritt* [2000] EHLR 24 and H&HI (6) 1; 5)).

The issue of "curtilage" and single curtilage is one that is sometimes raised. In *Cook v Minion* (1978) 37 P.& C.R 58, Walton J found that two separately occupied cottages built, built onto one another and owned by the same landlord were a single building and that water closets in the gardens serving the cottages were within the same curtilage. "Curtilage was an 'enclosure' or 'land within an enclosure'". Obviously, there must be some structures as to which the only reasonable conclusion is that they are "one building only". "On the other hand, there must be some structures that no reasonable tribunal could find to be "one building only". Between these two extremes, there will be many structures in respect of which there are conflicting criteria, some pointing to the structure being "one building", others to the contrary. As so often where there are conflicting criteria, which have to be weighed one against another, it is a question of fact whether a structure is on is not "one building". It should also be noted that building and house are not necessarily synonymous.

This was the view of the Court of Appeal based on examination of the authorities; *Hedley v. Webb* [1901] 2 Ch. 126; *Humphrey v. Young* [1903] 1 K.B. 44; 1 L.G.R. 142. Both these cases concerned semi-detached houses: in the former case, the pair was held on all the facts to be "one building" (though Cozens-Hardy J. made it clear that he was not saying that a pair of semi-detached houses were necessarily "one building"); in the latter case, the

Divisional Court refused to interfere with a finding of magistrates that the semi-detached houses in question were separate buildings".

Lord Simon Of Glaisdale in *Weaver v. Family Housing Association (York) Ltd.* House Of Lords 74 LGR 255, [1976] RA 25, [1976] EG 92 said that ... "although structural unity is undoubtedly a factor for consideration, I do not think that it can be ...conclusive,...... it would obviously be extravagant to suggest that every terrace of houses (from the countless ones constructed last century in industrial towns to Carlton House Terrace) must be "one building" because of structural unity. Many structures, which are unquestionably "one building", have more than one drainage outlet. On the other hand, there are premises that are undoubtedly separate buildings that have a common drainage system (see e.g., *Harris v. Scurfield* (1904) 2 L.G.R. 974)". The judgement continued, referring approvingly to *Harris v. Scurfield*, in which it was said that that case "concerned drainage by a common drain from an area embracing two blocks of back-to-back houses, a total of 18 houses. Although (unlike the instant case) there was common access by means of a court and certain facilities (such as ashpits and water closets) were in common, a Divisional Court of the King's Bench Division considered that the magistrates were not justified in holding that they were 'premises within the same curtilage'".

In this case, their Lordships also suggested matters that were relevant, although not all were given equal weight, these were:

* Structural unity
* Unity of ownership
* Occupation by separate tenants without intercommunication
* Existence of a single comprehensive system of drainage
* Separate cold stores
* Separate outside lavatories

In *St Martins-in-the-Field Vestry v Bird* [1895] 1 Q.B. 428, it was held that an arcade with a number of houses and shops on either side, roofed over and with gates at either end, was held not to be buildings or premises within the same curtilage.

Section 219 of the 1991 Act says that "drain" means a drain used for the drainage of one building or of any buildings or yards appurtenant to buildings within the same curtilage. The term 'sewer' is not actually defined precisely, although s.219 of the 1991 Act says that it includes "all sewers and drains (not being drains within the meaning given by this subsection) which are used for the drainage of buildings and yards appurtenant to buildings". The section goes on to say that any reference to the term pipe within the legislation, including references "to a main, a drain, or a sewer, shall include references to a tunnel or conduit that serves or is to serve as the pipe in question and to any accessories for the pipe".

As made clear in Garner [2], it has been and remains a fundamental principle of sewerage law, whether under Public Health Acts or the Water Industry Act, that sewers and drains should be designed so as to drain buildings and constructed objects such as roads, as distinct from land itself. It does not follow, however, that the "sewer" should carry sewage (*Ferrand v Hallas Land and Building Com*pany [1893] 2Q.B 135). The contents of the pipe do not determine whether it is a sewer, as it could carry rain or surface water.

That said, a watercourse does not become a sewer as a result of culverting (*George Legge & Son Ltd v Wenlock Corporation* [1936] 3 All ER 599, *British Railways Board v Tonbridge and Malling DC* (1981) 79 L.G.R 565 C.A., and *Sefton MBC v United Utilities Water Ltd* [2001] EWCA Civ 1284), although it is interesting that Bazalgette enclosed some of the tributaries of the Thames to form some of his sewer network for London. The issue of function is important, however, as at first instance in the *British Railways Board* case it had been held that the culvert was a sewer but not used "for the drainage of buildings". It should also be noted that s.262 of the Public Health Act 1936 gives power to a local authority to require culverting of watercourses and ditches where building operations are in prospect.

Where a sewer is constructed for the purposes of draining a number of premises, it is a "sewer" even if it in the end serves only one building at some point (*J. Pullan & Sons Ltd v Leeds City Council* (1990) 7 Constr.L.J. 222 C.A. and *Bromley LBC v Morritt* [2000] EHLR 24 C.A.). In the same way, a sewer designed for the drainage of a building does not cease to be a sewer just because it is not usable or not used at all – the "original purpose test" (*Blackdown Properties Ltd v Ministry of Housing and Local Government* [1967] 1 Ch 115.). In this case, a change of plan and work in developing a new estate left a length of sewer redundant and sealed off. Some years later, the local authority had made a declaration, vesting the whole of the sewer in itself. It was held that it was the function for which the pipe was constituted, not its actual use, that was important, and the sealed-off portion remained a "sewer".

A "sewer" must conduct effluent or liquid from one place to another and then discharge it. "It must have a terminus a quo and a terminus ad quem" (Buckley LJ. in *Pakenham v Ticehurst R.D.C.* (1903) 67 J.P. 448). On this construction, a line of pipes terminating in a cesspool (defined below) would not be a "sewer" as there is no discharge.

Until 2011, the distinction between a drain and a sewer had added significance, as the decision was then whether a sewer was a "public' or "private" sewer, that is, whether it was the responsibility of the WaSC or the collective responsibility of the owners of the properties served. This was changed as a result of amendments to the 1991 Act by the Water Act 2003 and the Water Industry (Schemes for Adoption of Private Sewers) Regulations 2011.[1] The result was that all private sewers became the responsibility of the WaSCs, and the notion of public lateral drains was also introduced, so that some drains also became the responsibility of the WaSCs. Subject to the rights of owners of private sewers, the WaSCs had a duty to transfer into their ownership by 1 October 2011 all sewers and lateral drains that had been connected to a public sewer before 1 July 2011, unless either the sewer or lateral drain was:

- owned by a railway undertaker; or
- located on Crown land, and the relevant authority (as defined by the regulations) has opted out of the scheme for transfer.

Sewerage companies had a duty to transfer pumping stations that form part of a private sewer or lateral drain no later than 1 October 2016.

Lateral drains and public laterals are discussed further below.

Aquifer

This is an underground layer of permeable rock, sediment, or soil that yields water. Aquifers can range from a few square kilometres to thousands of square kilometres in size. Geologically, this is a water-bearing bed or stratum, necessarily of some open-textured rock. Groundwater enters an aquifer as precipitation seeps through the soil. It can move through the aquifer and resurface through springs and wells. There are two general types of aquifers: confined and unconfined. Confined aquifers have a layer of impenetrable rock or clay above them, while unconfined aquifers lie below a permeable layer of soil [3].

Bathing waters (& directive)

A bathing water is a coastal or inland water that attracts a large number of bathers in relation to any infrastructure or facilities that are provided, or other measures that are taken, to promote bathing at the site. The UK has over 600 designated Bathing Waters, as reported by the outdoor swimming society [4][2]: sites that are popular for swimming and paddling and have been designated under the Bathing Water Regulations 2013.[3] They have been put in place as a result of the EU Bathing Waters Directive (2006/7/EC) in 1976. UK designated Bathing Waters are mostly coastal, with only 16 lakes, and two stretches of rivers in England and Wales have bathing water status as a result of local campaigns by those wishing to swim in the rivers. There are over 1,000 inland bathing waters in France [5]. There is no set limit for how many bathers are needed for a site to be identified as a bathing water.

A bathing water could be a coastal water in a large resort or a smaller site attracting a large number of bathers for its size.[4] However, it does not include every water where people swim and certainly not all waters where people undertake leisure activities. Designation can seem somewhat arbitrary given the "bathing season" and liable to "political" machinations.

Local councils must display information at the bathing water to show water quality during the bathing season (15 May to 30 September). Such bathing waters can be classified as 'excellent', 'good', 'sufficient', or 'poor'. Water Quality standards have been set for designated bathing waters based on World Health Organisation research into the incidence of stomach upsets in people bathing in waters with different levels of bacteria. Water is tested for two types of bacteria, *E. coli* and intestinal enterococci, as markers for sewage pollution.

It should be noted *Anglian Water Service Ltd v Environment Agency* [2020] EWHC 3544 (Admin), [2021] All ER (D) 24 (Jan), it was found in an action for judicial review the Environment Agency (EA) had misdirected itself in law in considering it had had no discretion to take account of an abnormal situation (heavy rainfall) in its assessment and classification of bathing water quality, in circumstances where the pollution source had not been known. Accordingly, the Administrative Court allowed, in part, Anglian Water Services Ltd's claim, challenging the EA's classification of the water quality at three popular beaches in Lincolnshire as 'good' (as opposed to 'excellent') in 2019.

It is interesting, given local authority's public health role, that "bathing prohibited" signs[5] are not used in England and Wales because this would require local authorities to close access to bathing water and enforce the prohibition. Defra has taken the view that merely providing advice against bathing was more proportionate.

Table 1.1 Total number of waters suitable for bathing in some EU countries in 2019, by country[a]

Country	Number
Italy	5,535
France	3,348
Germany	2,291
Spain	2,234
Greece	1,634
Denmark	1,022
Croatia	988
Netherlands	724
United Kingdom	644
Portugal	614
Poland	606
Sweden	438
Finland	301
Ireland	147

[a] https://www.statista.com/statistics/422323/ bathing-waters-in-europe-by-country/

Canal and River Trust

This body is responsible for the management of the 2,000-mile-long, 200-year-old, network of canals, rivers, reservoirs, and docks. In 2012, all of British Waterways' assets and responsibilities in England and Wales were transferred to this newly founded charity. In Scotland, British Waterways continues to operate as a standalone public corporation under the trading name Scottish Canals. Canals are "controlled waters".

Cesspool

This is a sealed underground tank that holds foul and waste water from a building (usually domestic properties). It should have no outlet and should be emptied by a tanker when full. The owner should record when the cesspool is emptied. These are usually found in rural areas and where it is not possible to install a septic tank. It was not unknown before prefabricated tanks were available for brick-built cesspools to have a hole knocked through after local authority inspection when installed. This would allow contents to escape, thus polluting the ground but avoiding the need for regular emptying but see s.50 Public Health Act 1936.

Chalk streams

Chalk streams are unique, with only about 200 in the world, and most of them are in the southern half of England (with a few in France). These streams emerge from the chalk aquifer, so the very pure water is rich in minerals and remains at a fairly constant temperature year-round. This good water quality supports many invertebrate and fish species, making them an important haven for wildlife, but such streams are vulnerable to sewage pollution and abstraction.

Coastal waters

This means surface water on the landward side of a line at a distance of one nautical mile on the seaward side from the nearest point of the baseline from which the breadth of territorial waters is measured, extending where appropriate up to the outer limit of transitional waters.

Combined sewer

This refers to a sewer that takes both foul and surface water – most constructions before the 1960s that were served by combined sewers. One exception would be in rural areas where septic tanks or cesspools were used. Sewers installed in the UK since the 1960s should be separate, with the raw sewage from homes and businesses going to foul drainage and the rainwater passing to different pipelines and to different places. Raw sewage should go to treatment, and surface water may go to a surface water source such as a river or a soakaway.

There are around 100,000 km of combined sewers in England,[6] taking both foul and surface water, and in times of heavy rainfall increase the flow to a rate greater than sewage treatment works can cope with.

The Jenkins report [6] on the review of the arrangements for determining responsibility for surface water and drainage assets recommended that Defra re-examine the workings of Section 106 of the Water Industry Act of 1991 so as to ensure that the sewerage system is not subjected to unnecessary flood risk through the connection of surface water drainage. That is, combined sewers should not be the norm where there is a risk of flooding (see also below on sustainable urban drainage systems (SuDS)).

This term should not be confused with "drainage in combination", a term seen in older texts that refers to buildings drained in combination, which now makes that pipeline, when it collects sewage or water from the second building, a sewer.

Combined sewer overflow (outfall) (CSO) or storm overflows

These can be seen as safety valves built into the combined sewer system and are a problem resulting from combined sewers. They discharge excess sewage and rainwater to rivers, lakes, or the sea when the sewer system is supposedly under strain, that is, the capacity of the sewers is exceeded. This theoretically is intended to protect properties from flooding and prevent sewage from backing up into streets and homes during heavy storm events. The original idea is that the amount of rainwater causing the CSO to discharge means the sewage is diluted to the extent that it poses no risk to public health or the environment. As the paper from Giakoumis and Voulvoulis [7] says, CSOs are used to protect the works under peak dry weather flow conditions. Such frequent, and in some cases independent of rainfall, use of CSOs could have detrimental effects for the receiving environment as well as put thousands of water users at risk.

As the CMO for England and the chairs of the EA and Ofwat have said [8]

> *the engineering logic of storm overflows is that if the sewerage system is at risk of being overwhelmed by storms or atypically intense rain, sewers get too full and can back up into homes or overflow into streets. To prevent that, storm overflows act as a safety release valve, but were intended only for exceptional circumstances when the public would be unlikely to be using rivers.*

Table 1.2 Number of CSOs and duration of spills in 2022

Water company	No CSOs	Total no. Spills (events)	Total duration of spills (hrs)
Anglian Water	1,552	16,082	89,514
Dwr Cymru	126	2,800	9,470
Northumbrian Water	1,564	29,697	107,536
Severn Trent	2,466	44,765	249,116
South West	1,342	37,649	290,271
Southern Water	978	16,688	146,819
Thames Water	777	8,014	74,693
United Utilities	2,254	69,245	425,491
Wessex Water	1,300	21,878	129,957
Yorkshire Water	2,221	54,273	232,054
Total	14,580	301,091	1,754,921

Source: Environment Agency.

This whole approach and the issues arising from CSOs are discussed later below, as it is somewhat complacent as it is now clear that CSOs operate more frequently than they should, and it is these discharges that have caused such public concern in recent times. Public concern has been highlighted by the problems of sewage discharges onto beaches and the aquatic environment, including rivers used for wild swimming.

According to Government figures, there are approximately 15,000 CSO.s in England, and in 2020, there were over 400,000 sewage discharges totalling over three million hours. The latest figures are included in Table 1.2. There are around 15,000 storm overflows in England, and in 2020 there were over 400,000 sewage discharges, totalling over three million hours. In Wales, there are about 3,000 CSO.s, and there were 106,094 discharges from CSOs across the 3,700 km of sewer network. In the UK as a whole, there are said to be a total of 20,233 CSO.s. The BBC has suggested that if a member of the public has concerns over a discharge of sewage, they should raise them with "your local council or local water company, the EA, or a group like the Marine Conservation Society (MCS)".[7]

In March 2022, the Government issued a consultation on the "Storm Overflows Discharge Reduction Plan". The outcome of this proposal is discussed further in Chapter 5.

Consumer Council for Water

Consumer Council for Water is an independent voice for water consumers in England and Wales. Established under the Water Act 2003, it has helped consumers resolve complaints against their water company or retailer while providing free advice and support. They exist to champion the interests of consumers, influence water companies, governments, and regulators, and carry out research as well as investigate complaints.

The fourth "Testing the Waters" report published in January 2023[8] (the reports are published every two years) looks at how business customers in England and Wales feel about the water, sewerage, and retail services. This found overall satisfaction has declined for both water and sewerage services – from 91% to 88% and from 88% to 82%, respectively.

Controlled water

Section 104 of the Water Resources Act 1991 defines this as relevant territorial waters, which are waters extending seaward for three miles from the baselines from which the breadth of the territorial sea adjacent to England and Wales is measured plus coastal waters (waters that are within the area that extends landward from those baselines as far as the limit of the highest tide plus the waters of any relevant river or watercourse, the fresh-water limit of the river or watercourse, together with the waters of any enclosed dock that adjoins waters within that area). It also includes inland freshwaters, including canals, lakes, and ponds and groundwater.

Critical sewers

This is a term that was used by WaSCs and Ofwat, though it appears to have less importance to Ofwat than previously. It refers to those public sewers, which in the event of failure, would incur high costs in terms of repair and traffic delays. It also refers to those sewers that are considered to be strategically important. It was a means of trying to organise priorities for inspection via CCTV (or otherwise), investment, and renovation of the network. Using published Ofwat figures in 2009, the author calculated that at the rate of renewal or renovation of these sewers, the implied asset life ranged from 220 years for one WaSC to 1,114 for another. At that time, it was estimated that there were about 310,000 km of public sewers in the network, of which 73,537 are "critical".[9]

Dry-weather flow

This is the average daily flow to a sewage treatment works (WWTW) during a period without rain. The flow in a combined sewerage system will increase when it rains, and this may vary due to changing levels of sewer infiltration and population numbers (see also peak wet weather flow and peak dry weather flow).

Environment Agency (EA) (SEPA and other regulators)

The EA is an executive, non-departmental public body sponsored by the Department for Environment, Food & Rural Affairs (Defra). Within England, the EA is responsible for regulating major industry and waste, the treatment of contaminated land, water quality and resources, fisheries, inland river, estuary, and harbour navigation, conservation, and ecology. The EA is also responsible for managing the risk of flooding from main rivers, reservoirs, estuaries, and the sea.

Lead local flood authorities are county councils and unitary authorities with responsibility for managing the risk of flooding from surface water, groundwater, and ordinary watercourses and leading community recovery.

In Scotland, the Scottish Environment Protection Agency (SEPA) is a non-departmental public body of the Scottish Government. Its role is to make sure that the environment and human health are protected, to ensure that Scotland's natural resources and services are used as sustainably as possible, and to con-tribute to sustainable economic growth.

In Wales, Natural Resources Wales fulfils the same functions as the EA in England and is the environmental regulator with a role to monitor discharges.

The Northern Ireland Environment Agency has as its primary purpose the protection and enhancement of Northern Ireland's environment, and in doing so, deliver health and well-being benefits and supports economic growth. The Agency's key priorities are a fully compliant regulated industry, a freshwater and marine environment at "good status", a compliant crime-free waste sector, good habitat and landscape quality with species abundance and diversity, and the promotion of environmentally sustainable development and infrastructure.

Eutrophication and eutrophic waters

Eutrophication is seen as a leading cause of impairment in many freshwater and coastal marine ecosystems around the world. Eutrophication is character-ised by excessive plant and algal growth due to the enrichment of the water by nutrients, particularly nitrogen and/or phosphorous, as can be found in fertilis-ers and sewage, leading to the rapid growth of algae and other plant forms. Although over many years this will occur naturally, human activities have accelerated the rate and extent of eutrophication through both point-source discharges and non-point loadings of limiting nutrients. Such an acceleration can have dramatic consequences for drinking water sources, fisheries, and recreational water bodies [9]. Eutrophic water is where eutrophication is well advanced in a body of water. Eutrophication was intended to be addressed via the Urban Wastewater Treatment Directive.[10]

Exfiltration

This is the term used to describe the leakage of wastewater out of a sewer-age system through broken or damaged pipes and manholes. Wastewater that leaks out of defective pipe joints and cracks can contaminate groundwater and surface water. Other problems can include structural failures when the soil and supporting material for the pipeline are eroded, which can lead to subsidence of the pipeline and breakage or distortion that affects the flow.

Sewers may vary between exfiltration and infiltration (see below) depending on groundwater conditions. A study reported in Barrett et al. [10] using marker species indicated that pollution of the shallow aquifer as a result of exfiltration was widespread. It was concluded that the sources were leaky lateral pipes rather than main sewers, which would be below the water table; it is these pipes that local authority environmental health officers could deal with, and the legal basis for this is addressed later in the book.

Exfiltration has environmental impacts but also has the effect of reducing the flow in the sewers and will not contribute to sewer flooding or discharges from combined sewer outfalls. That said, infiltration and exfiltration are two sides of the same coin, and which occurs will depend on the level of the water table or even the proximity and condition of water supply pipes.

External flooding

In the context of sewers, external flooding is defined as flooding within the curtilage of a building normally used for residential, public, community, and business purposes.

Flow to Full Treatment (FFT)

This is a measure of how much wastewater a treatment works must be able to treat at any time. They should be able to deal with a certain amount of wastewater, calculated depending on the area they serve, and many have a requirement in their environmental permit about the Flow to Full Treatment (FFT) level they must work to. If the amount of wastewater going to the works is more than the FFT level, for example, if there is a storm and heavy rain, then the environmental permit for the treatment works will normally allow the extra amount coming into the works to be diverted to storm tanks (where the works has them) until the storm passes. The contents of these storm tanks can then be returned to be treated by the works.

If the storm is prolonged or sustained, the environmental permits will allow the water company to release the extra incoming rainwater and diluted wastewater into the environment, normally after partial treatment. This is considered further later, in particular how the permitting regime has led to increased sewage pollution.

If a water company is diverting this rain and wastewater to storm tanks or the environment before reaching the works' FFT level, they could be breaking the conditions of their environmental permit.

Fats, Oil, and Grease (FOG)

Fat, oil, and grease deposits (FOG) in sewers are a major problem and can cause sewer overflows, resulting in environmental damage and health risks. There appears to be a complex reaction in the sewer, particularly with detergents. It has been simplistically portrayed as the cooling of fats, but recent research has suggested that saponification may be involved in FOG formation [11].

FOG generated from commercial food service establishments can form hardened solids, and it has been estimated that these are responsible for approximately 50–75% of annual sanitary sewer overflows in the USA [12] (no equivalent figure is available for the UK).

Forever chemicals

Per- and polyfluoroalkyl substances (PFAS) are commonly referred to as "forever chemicals" as they do not breakdown in the environment (the EU is considering a ban) as not only are they persistent but pose a threat to health. They are widespread in drinking water in the USA.[11] The House of Commons Environmental Audit Committee reported that one chemical in this family, PFOS, is prohibited under the 2009 Stockholm Convention on Persistent Organic Pollutants, but despite this, in 465 samples taken between 2014 and 2018, 46% of English rivers failed the Water Framework Directive threshold for PFOS.43. "This underlines its persistence in the environment" [13].

The chemicals have been used in tens of thousands of products. PFASs are widely used in stain repellents, paints and polishes. cars, textiles, medical gear, and non-stick pans due to their long-term resistance to extreme temperatures and corrosion. They can get into surface water as a result of run-off from construction sites, roads, and surface water drainage around homes (which are not monitored or effectively regulated), as well as via domestic sewage and wastewater treatment works.

Grey water

This is wastewater other than that from a toilet or other sanitary installation and is produced by domestic processes. It has a relatively low level of contamination. This includes wastewater being drained from sinks or the used water that's pumped out of a washing machine.

While greywater is not suitable for human consumption, it can be used, for example, for watering the garden. There are greywater recycling systems that help reduce water consumption, and these can be used for irrigation systems, flushing toilets, and even washing clothes.

Groundwater

This is water that has dropped as precipitation and that has then infiltrated the ground to fill the spaces between sediments and cracks in rock. Groundwater is fed by precipitation and can resurface to replenish streams, rivers, and lakes. It fills in the empty spaces underground, in the saturated zone, until it reaches an impenetrable layer of rock. Groundwater is contained and flows through bodies of rock and sediment, which are aquifers (see above). The top of the saturated zone is the water table, and sitting above the water table is the unsaturated zone, where the spaces in between rocks and sediments are filled with both water and air. This is soil moisture and is distinct from groundwater. Groundwater can be discharged through springs, lakes, rivers, streams, or manmade wells. It is recharged by precipitation, snowmelt, or water seepage from other sources, including irrigation and leaks from water supply systems or sewers, so that leaking sewers (exfiltration) can pollute groundwater. Groundwater can enter a defective sewer or drain as infiltration (see below). The direction of flow may reflect the height of the water table and can vary between exfiltration and infiltration as the water table varies.

Highway drain

These are drains that take surface water that drains from roads and footpaths and then flows into public sewerage systems. For the purposes of s.100 of the Highways Act 1980, a 'highway drain' is defined as including a ditch, gutter, watercourse, soak-away, bridge, culvert, tunnel, or pipe. However, to be such a drain, it must have been constructed for the purpose of carrying away surface water from a road. A 'highway drain' will not be a sewer as it is not used for the drainage of buildings and yards, but it may become one if its functions include the drainage of such premises.

Drains that take surface water from a highway and that serve no other purpose will normally be vested in the highway authority by s.263 of the Highways Act 1980. This is usually the County Council or metropolitan districts outside London; the main exceptions are trunk and special roads vested in the Secretary of State (Highways Agency). A drain on the highway is the responsibility of the highway authority only if it is not a public sewer, forms part of the road or highway, or is vested in the highway authority.

House of commons select committees

The Environmental Audit Committee's remit is to consider the extent to which the policies and programmes of government departments and non-departmental public bodies contribute to environmental protection and sustainable development and to audit their performance against sustainable development and environmental protection targets. Unlike most select committees, the

Committee's remit cuts across government rather than focussing on the work of a particular department. The Committee also receives support from the National Audit Office.

Environment, Food and Rural Affairs Committee is a select committee that scrutinises the administration, spending, and policy of the Government's Department for Environment, Food, and Rural Affairs.

Infiltration

The progressive degradation of the structural state of urban sewerage systems leads to the presence of tightness defects, which, depending on the level of the groundwater table or on the water content in the sewer trenches, can generate two phenomena, one of which is infiltration [10] (the other is exfiltration). Infiltration is the term used to describe the entry of freshwater, or groundwater, into sewer systems through defects or damage in pipes or joints, manholes, or inspection access points. Infiltration can also include an inflow of flow from storm water runoff and groundwater that enters sewer systems. Leaking water supply pipes can add to the rate of infiltration. This all adds to the flow within the sewer and therefore to the flow of sewage to the treatment works There are several methods of measuring infiltration rates [14].

In a report for the Campaign for the Renewal of Older Sewers (CROSS) [10], it was reported that a study in the Lambourne Valley in Berkshire found high infiltration volumes. Indeed, that work concluded there were infiltration rates of 75–82% of the total sewage flow in an average year. The degree of infiltration bore a strong correlation with groundwater levels. As a result of a sewer sealing programme, there were much reduced pumping costs as the flow in the sewer was also reduced. Work by CIRIA [15] indicated that 28% of sewer catchments had greater than 25% infiltration and 9% more than 50%, and infiltration was a major cause of overload of the treatment work and pumping stations and premature operation of the CSOs in a number of catchments.

Internal flooding

In the context of sewers, internal flooding is defined as flooding that enters a building or passes below a suspended floor.

Lateral drain (and public lateral)

A lateral drain means those parts of a drain that run from (outside) the curtilage of a building (or buildings or yards within the same curtilage) to the sewer with which the drain communicates or is to communicate. "Curtilage" is discussed in the context of what is a sewer above; the amendments to the legislation that introduced the idea of "public laterals" did not clarify the term but left it to guidance as the legislation made provision for the transfer of laterals to WaSCs. Thus, there are "public lateral drains", i.e., lateral drains that either belong to the sewerage undertaker or are vested in the sewerage undertaker by virtue of a declaration made under Section 102 of the 1991 Act above or under an agreement made under Section 104 of the 1991 Act.

As of 2004, new laterals may not be connected to a public sewer unless they are built to an adoptable standard, and adoption agreements may require inspection chambers (demarcation chambers) to be constructed to an adoptable standard close to the curtilage of the property to act as a demarcation point between the drain from the property (which remains the householder's responsibility) and the lateral (which becomes the sewerage undertaker's responsibility).

Figures 1.1A and 1.1B below are taken from guidance that illustrates where responsibility lies, but there may well be some circumstances that do not fully match these scenarios.

Leisure waters

This is not a legal term but is used to describe any water where people undertake leisure activities. It may be natural or artificial and can be used to describe water systems other than designated Bathing Waters.

As Pond and Bond have said in Clay's 22nd Edn [16], the requirements for preventing and responding to recreational water illnesses can vary significantly amongst local and state agencies. In the UK, there are no specific regulations governing the design, construction, and management of swimming pool facilities other than provisions of the Health and Safety at Work, etc. Act 1974.[12] There are no controls at all over the quality of other leisure waters (unless also designated as Bathing Waters) other than general environmental or pollution controls.

The reality is, as the CMO for England et al. have said,

> use of our rivers for recreation and exercise is something to celebrate and encourage. Children have always played in waterways and always will, irrespective of what notices are put up next to them. People of all ages use freshwater waterways such as rivers for recreation including swimming and various forms of boating. During lockdown many people took to swimming in rivers and have continued since. Our rivers, seas and waterways should therefore be free from sewage to reduce risk to the public.

Marine Conservation Society (MCS)

The MCS is a UK-based not-for-profit organisation that campaigns for a cleaner, better-protected, and healthier ocean. It works with businesses,

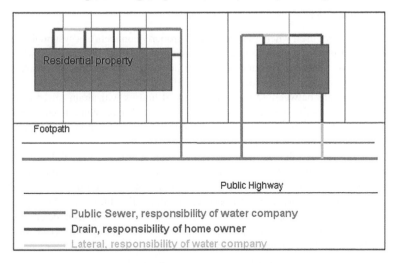

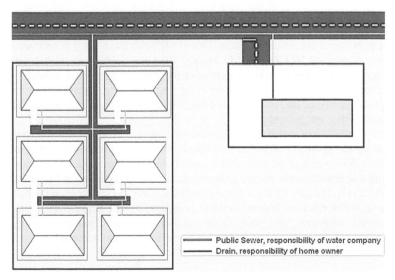

Figure 1.1 (A) Arrangements of responsibilities following the transfer of private sewers to WaSCs (simple illustration for individual properties). (B) Arrangements of responsibilities following the transfer of private sewers to WaSCs (simple illustration for apartment blocks)

governments, and communities to clean and protect the oceans and beaches, campaigns to stop pollution entering the oceans, and organises volunteer beach cleans to remove and record the litter on the UK's coastline.[13]

Misconnection

This is a term used when drainage from a property connects to a system that is inappropriate for the wastewater that is being discharged. For example, when a domestic appliance is connected to a surface water drain that then discharges into a river, stream, or soakaway. In the UK, the Rivers Trust[14] is estimated that there are between 150,000 and 500,000 houses with drain misconnections. This is often caused by faulty plumbing and inadequate investigation before installations are put in after the completion of the house. It is more common in older properties.

It is estimated that 15% of rivers in England and Wales have failed water quality standards because of misconnections, thus creating a risk to the ecosystem and public health. Rivers can become contaminated by sewage and dangerous chemicals used in household products like bleach and shampoo, posing a threat to plant and animal life. Where a toilet is misconnected, this could result in items flushed away, including tampons and wet wipes (see non-flushable products), ending up in watercourses.

National Infrastructure Commission (NIC)

The National Infrastructure Commission (NIC) was established as an Executive Agency of HM Treasury in January 2017 and operates at arm's length from the government. The objectives of the NIC are to support sustainable economic growth across all regions of the UK, improve competitiveness, improve quality of life, and support climate resilience and the transition to net zero carbon emissions by 2050.[15]

The NIC has called for stricter controls on new property developments alongside up to £12 billion of investment in drainage infrastructure over the next thirty years to stop thousands more homes and businesses from flooding due to inadequate drainage, according to a report published in November 2022 [17]. In high-risk areas, local authorities, water and sewerage companies, and, where relevant, internal drainage boards, should be required to develop costed, long-term joint plans to manage surface water flooding, including local targets for risk reduction assured by the EA with input from Ofwat.

Non-flushable products

Non-flushable products are those products and materials that should not be flushed down the toilet because of the risks to the sewerage infrastructure, including treatment works. Baby wipes, wet wipes (used for many tasks from make-up removal to surface cleaning), and other non-flushable materials can block sewers and cost customers and water and sewerage companies millions of pounds a year in cleaning and repairs. A study in New York identified flushed products found at two pump station inlet screens at Ward Island; one from the Bronx and one from Manhattan. The study found that 98% of the contents were non-flushable products such as baby wipes, hygiene products, and paper [18].

In 2018, the BBC reported that all wet wipes sold as "flushable" in the UK had so far failed the water industry's disintegration tests. Water companies say wet wipes don't break down and are causing blockages that cost millions to put right. Manufacturers insist their test is adequate and say sewer blockages are caused by people putting non-flushable wipes down the toilet.[16]

Even if ultimate responsibility for sewage discharges and CSOs operating too frequently falls to the WaSCs, the management of sewerage systems is made more difficult by plastic wet wipes flushed down toilets, which congeal together with fats poured down drains to form "fatbergs", blocking sewers, restricting flows, and causing avoidable use of the storm overflows.

Office for Environmental Protection

Established by the Environment Act 2021, it has the purpose of protecting and improving the environment by holding the government and public authorities, including regulators, local authorities, and water companies (in respect of their public powers and duties), to account so far as environmental performance is concerned. The work includes monitoring the implementation of environmental law, advising the government on environmental law to comply with environmental law and enforcing against failures (it will receive complaints about failures of compliance). Its powers and duties are set out in the 2021 Act.

Ofwat

The Water Services Regulation Authority is a non-ministerial government department established in 1989, when the water and sewerage industry in England and Wales was privatised. Under Section 2 of WIA91 as amended, Ofwat must carry out most of our work as an economic regulator in the way we consider best and "further the consumer objective to protect the interests of consumers, wherever appropriate, by promoting effective competition". It also has responsibility for ensuring that WaSCs properly carry out their statutory functions. It has also to secure that water companies can (in particular by securing reasonable returns on their capital) finance the proper carrying out of their statutory functions. Ofwat has responsibility for ensuring that water supply licensees and sewerage licensees properly carry out their licensed activities and statutory functions.

It also has to ensure the long-term resilience of water companies' water supply and wastewater systems and secure that they take steps to enable them, in the long term, to meet the need for water supplies and wastewater services. While the EA is the main body responsible for regulating water quality and ecological protection, Ofwat should play a key role in driving and enabling the water sector to protect and improve the environment. This means that Ofwat should, as part of the price review process, ensure adequate investment in environmental initiatives and ensure water companies deliver environmental improvements. It is a moot point as to how effective Ofwat is in ensuring adequate investment in the sewerage infrastructure.

Oligotrophic waters

These are water bodies (rivers and lakes) that are lacking plant nutrients and have a large amount of dissolved oxygen throughout. In rivers, these are typically those that have a rapid flow and stony beds. An oligotroph is an organism that can live in an environment that offers very low levels of nutrients, in contrast to copiotrophs, which prefer nutritionally rich environments. Oligotrophs are characterised by slow growth, low rates of metabolism, and generally low population density and are adapted such that they will not survive in nutrient-rich environments, such as those where sewage and agricultural pollution run off into such wasters. Fish of the Salmonidae, such as trout, can be found in oligotrophic waters and will suffer where there is a change in water quality.

Peak dry weather flow

This term is used interchangeably with "dry weather flow" in the UK, and sewage (wastewater) treatment works should be designed to treat peak dry weather flow and additional flows from light rainfall. A dry day is a day when rainfall does not exceed 0.25 mm.

Peak wet weather flow

This is the combined flow of sewage and stormwater in wet weather and can be used to calculate the level when sewage treatment or wastewater treatment works cannot cope and need to bypass secondary treatment processes, that is, when wet weather event flows exceed the capacity of the treatment plant and risk damage to the treatment process. A WaSC should design, construct, and maintain sewerage systems (including CSOs) according to best technical knowledge not entailing excessive cost and limit pollution from storm overflows. As ever, it is the NEEC that is the contentious part.

Public sewer

These are sewers, which are the responsibility of the sewerage undertaking. How sewers become public sewers is discussed further in Chapter 3.

Public lateral drain (or public lateral)

See above on *Lateral drains.*

Pumping station

In most circumstances, gravity is what causes sewage to flow down a pipeline. In low-lying areas where the main sewer sits on higher ground than the domestic sewage pipes and where the "fall" or gradient cannot be achieved, the sewage needs to be transported in a different way. Sewage will then sit in the well until it reaches a predetermined level. A pumping station is made up of a large tank, known as a wet well, that acts as the receiver for sewage from a building or buildings. Once it reaches this level, a pump will cut in to pressurise the sewage so that it can then travel from the wet well uphill to a point where it can enter a sewer that has an adequate fall and can then be used for the sewage to flow to treatment.

Private pumping stations that serve more than one property were also subject to transfer to the WaSCs, and this happened in 2016.

River Action

Launched in 2021, River Action is a campaigning organisation with a mission to rescue Britain's rivers by raising awareness about river pollution and applying pressure on industrial and agricultural producers, water companies, and other polluters. The most high-profile member of the campaign is Feargal Sharkey.[17] The aim is to make the industry take greater responsibility for remedying the adverse environmental impact their supply chains are having on the health of our rivers. Since its launch, River Action has led a number of high-profile campaigns that have increased public awareness of the pollution crisis facing our rivers and the failure of Government-funded environmental agencies to address it.

Rivers Trust

This is an umbrella organisation of 65 member River Trusts in the UK and Ireland. Local Trusts work to achieve positive improvements in river quality and stop pollution. The organisation has expertise in river and catchment quality and conservation.[18]

Septic tank

This is a small treatment system that is not connected to the main sewer system and is most commonly used in rural areas. The tanks contain bacteria that break down organic waste. The inclusion of a bacterial treatment mechanism is the difference between a septic tank and a cesspool.

Installed underground, a septic tank makes use of natural processes to treat the sewage it stores. Usually made up of two chambers or compartments, the tank receives wastewater from an inlet pipe. These days, most septic tanks are pre-formed package systems.

Little maintenance is required, but frequent de-sludging is important to ensure a buildup does not occur, and solids should be removed from the tank annually. It is even more important than for the public sewerage system that certain items are not put in the drains that serve the septic tank as they can block the inlet or inhibit bacterial activity. These include food waste, fat, oil, and grease, plastic bags, nappies and sanitary products, pharmaceuticals, and cleaning wipes.

Sewage

See above, and means the contents of the sewerage system. The contents of sewage and why it poses a threat to both public health and the environment are dealt with in Chapter 2.

Sewage sludge

Sewage or wastewater treatment is considered a way of preventing contaminants from reaching the environment (see below), but the solid material left from treatment is sewage sludge. This sludge, once treated, can spread on agricultural land as it contains high levels of nutrients such as nitrogen and phosphorus and is a source of organic matter, but it can also contain microplastics and per- and PFAS, the so-called "forever chemicals" because they do not degrade in the environment (see above). In the UK, treated sludge is estimated to contain 69–80% of the microplastics that enter treatment works. While the water is cleaned and discharged, the remaining toxic sewage sludge stays at the treatment plant and has been described as "the most pollutant-rich manmade substance on Earth".[19]

This "biosolid" sludge is expensive to dispose of because it must be landfilled, but the waste management industry is increasingly using a money-making alternative: repackaging the sludge as fertiliser and injecting it into the nation's food chain. It is argued that the practice is behind a growing number of public health problems. Spreading pollutant-filled biosolids on farmland is causing illness [19].

Sewage treatment

Sewage treatment plants, sometimes called wastewater treatment plants, are installations to treat sewage and remove contaminants and pollutants so that an effluent is produced that can be safely discharged into the environment.

Treatment is usually biological but with physical aspects; the steps are pre-treatment to remove coarse materials and screening to remove large objects that can be found in sewage, such as rags, non-flushable products, sticks, and plastic containers. The next stage is grit removal and heavier materials via settlement. There may also be flow equalisation with the intention of reducing peak dry-weather flows or peak wet-weather flows where there are combined sewer systems. There may also be a stage involving fat and grease removal. Primary treatment is the removal of suspended solids and other organic matter, where sewage passes through a container where other solids can settle out and oil and grease can float to the top and be skimmed off. Secondary treatment removes most of the other solids using biological processes to digest and remove this material and uses aerobic or anaerobic processes to reduce the biological oxygen demand. Tertiary treatment can include disinfection, biological nutrient removal, and the removal of micro-pollutants, including pharmaceutical pollutants. Treated effluent is sometimes disinfected chemically or physically, such as by lagoons and microfiltration, prior to discharge. The solids are what make up sewage sludge, which is further treated.

Sewerage

See above on the difference between sewerage (the infrastructure) and sewage (the contents).

Soakaway

A soakaway is a hole dug into the ground that is filled with coarse stone and rubble in layers or plastic crates. It allows water to filter through it, and literally and soak steadily into the ground. Soakaways are used to manage surface water at their source and serve as an alternative to draining off surface water via a stream or sewer system. They can be an effective way of dealing with relatively small amounts of surface water from, for example, a small roof.

Soakaways collect all surface water run-off at one point before allowing it to percolate in a controlled manner into the surrounding ground/earth in the area where it falls. Some modern soakaways are created using 'soakaway crates' that allow the water to filter through in exactly the same manner. Whether a soakaway is appropriate depends on the ground conditions. The soil around the hole should be granular and be able to effectively drain away the excess water, so it is unsuitable for clay areas.

Surfers against Sewage[20]

Based in Cornwall, it began in 1990 as a response by the surfing community to the state of the beaches and sewage pollution. Those hardy souls who ventured into the water back then often found themselves swimming in raw sewage. In 2012, Surfers Against Sewage was recognised as a national marine conservation charity focused on the protection of waves, oceans, beaches, marine wildlife, and coastal communities. More recently, SoS has campaigned against plastic pollution of the seas.

Sustainable Urban Drainage (SuDS)

SuDS have been developed to improve drainage and reduce the volume of surface runoff in urban areas. The use of green space in the design of SuDS allows water to be controlled using trees and vegetation, green roofs, ponds, and wetlands. Green roofs can especially be implemented in order to increase interception, storm water storage, and evaporation in highly urbanised areas where the space to introduce green infrastructure is restricted.[21]

Alongside a reduction in the risk of flooding, SuDS in the urban landscape can also provide other environmental and ecological benefits. The inclusion of green space within SUDS can also contribute to noise reduction, air filtering, and provide an aesthetically pleasing communal green space. Furthermore, green roofs have been found to support a wide variety of insects and birds, and wetlands can support aquatic species.

The Local Government Association [20] has said SuDS essentially operate through infiltration where possible and attenuation combined with slow conveyance. Many SuDS solutions employ a combination of infiltration and attenuation. Situations where infiltration is not an option, for example, because of the soil type or contamination, tend to favour attenuation-type SuDS.

SuDS design should adhere to a number of key principles:

- Using a number of SuDS components in series and characterising areas by land use and drainage type
- Managing runoff as close as possible to where it falls as rain
- Managing water on the surface – wherever possible, runoff should be managed on the surface
- Early and effective engagement – consider the use of SuDS at the earliest stages of site selection and design

In England, Schedule 3 of the Flood and Water Management Act 2010 was not commenced, as the government sought to increase the use of SuDS through planning policy from April 2015. Current planning policy requires that SuDS be included in all new major developments (developments over ten homes), unless there is clear evidence that this would be inappropriate. This is in addition to the requirement that SuDS should be given priority in new developments in flood-risk areas. However, as Defra conceded in January 2023, the planning route has been found not to be effective. Schedule 3 provides a framework for the approval and adoption of drainage systems, an approving body, and national standards on the design, construction, operation, and maintenance of SuDS. Also, it makes the right to connect surface water runoff to public sewers conditional upon the drainage system being approved before any construction work can start. The benefits of SuDs can only be realised if they are designed, constructed, adopted, and maintained to national standards for the lifetime of the development. The Government says that implementing Schedule 3 will guarantee this is achieved.

Trade effluent discharge

In the context of this book, trade effluent is any liquid waste, excluding domestic sewage and surface water, that is discharged from premises being used for a business, trade, or industrial process. Trade effluent can come from both large and small premises, including businesses such as car washes and launderettes. It can be effluent from an industrial or business process that is discharged into a public sewer, washed down a sink or toilet, or put into a private sewer that connects to the public sewer.

Without exception, the occupier of any trade premises in the area of a sewerage undertaker may only discharge trade effluent from their premises into the undertaker's public sewers with the consent of the undertaker (WaSC). A trade effluent consent is issued under the provisions of s.118 of the Water Industry Act 1991. It is an offence to discharge trade effluent without consent. The conditions attached to the consent will be such as to ensure the treatment works of the sewerage system are not adversely affected by the discharge.

Trade effluent may be wastewater contaminated with materials such as:

- fats, oils, and greases
- chemicals
- detergents
- heavy metal rinses
- solids
- food wastes

Macerated food waste is banned from sewers in most cases in Scotland and Northern Ireland.

The Trade Effluents (Prescribed Process and Substances) Regulations 1989,[22] amended in 1990 and 1992, specify a number of processes and substances as 'special category'. The relevant EA will have to be consulted and can either refuse the 'special category' discharge (prohibiting the discharge) or serve a Notice of Determination jointly on the WaSC and the customer requiring that certain conditions are not exceeded, and they will be included in the trade effluent discharge consent.

Urban wastewater

Council Directive 91/271/EEC concerning urban wastewater treatment was adopted on 21 May 1991 to protect the water environment from the adverse effects of discharges of urban wastewater and from certain industrial discharges. 'urban wastewater' means domestic wastewater or the mixture of domestic wastewater with industrial wastewater and/or run-off rainwater.

Vacuum sewerage system

Vacuum or pneumatic sewerage systems are used in a variety of situations where it is difficult to install a traditional gravity system, such as in low-lying areas and/or a high water table, or where there is an environmental issue, such as where there is an inadequate septic tank system or a failing cesspool. The main components of a vacuum sewer system are a collection chamber and vacuum valve, the pipeline, a central vacuum station, and monitoring and control elements. The system maintains a partial vacuum with air pressure below atmospheric inside the pipe network and vacuum station collection chamber. It rapidly transports sewage in a network of empty pipes from the collection chamber to a central collection tank and then to a treatment works. A pulse of sewage enters the vacuum system when the pneumatic valve opens in a collection chamber and the sewage is transported into the vacuum main. The valve remains open briefly following the removal of the sewage from the collection tank, allowing atmospheric air to enter the suction pipe and send the sewage onward.

Water UK

Water UK is a membership body representing the UK water industry, and members include all WaSCs across England, Wales, Scotland, and Northern Ireland. It also has a number of associate members who provide services outside the UK. It was established in 1998 to form a single voice for the water industry across the UK, bringing together the previous Water Services Association and Water Companies Association. It should be remembered that there are water-only companies (what were known as statutory water companies) that do not provide sewerage services.

Water Research Centre (WRc)

Initially created in 1927 as the Water Pollution Research Board for the government, the organisation evolved to undertake a growing number of research projects covering all aspects of water and wastewater supply, treatment, and catchment management. Water Research Centre (WRc) was privatised at the same time as the water industry in 1989 and has since operated as an independent consultancy. In 2020, WRc became part of the RSK Group, an integrated environmental, engineering, and technical services company.

Notes

1 SI 201No 1566.
2 The Outdoor Swimming Society was established in 2006 to pioneer outdoor swimming in rivers, lakes, lido and seas.
3 SI 2013 No 1675.
4 The list of designated bathing waters can be found at https://www.gov.uk/government/publications/bathing-waters-list-of-designated-waters-in-england/list-of-current-bathing-waters-2019-bathing-season
5 See https://www.gov.uk/guidance/bathing-water-information-and-signage-rules-for-local-councils#display-information
6 https://lordslibrary.parliament.uk/sewage-pollution-in-englands-waters/
7 http://news.bbc.co.uk/panorama/hi/front_page/newsid_8236000/8236957.stm
8 https://www.ccw.org.uk/publication/testing-the-waters-2022/
9 Included in notes for training course "The Legal Implications of Drains and Sewers" delivered by author.
10 91/271/EEC.
11 https://www.scientificamerican.com/article/forever-chemicals-are-widespread-in-u-s-drinking-water/
12 http://www.hse.gov.uk/legislation/hswa.htm
13 https://www.mcsuk.org
14 https://theriverstrust.org/about-us/news/drain-misconnections
15 See the charter for the NIC at https://assets.publishing.service.gov.uk/government/uploads/system/uploads/attachment_data/file/1028250/Updated_NIC_charter_v.final2.pdf.
16 https://www.bbc.co.uk/news/uk-46188354
17 Feargal Sharkey OBE is a singer most widely known as the lead vocalist of punk band The Undertones. A lifelong fly fisherman he has campaigned against the pollution of British rivers (particularly chalk streams) and is the Chairman of the Amwell Magna Fishery.
18 More information is at https://theriverstrust.org
19 https://www.theguardian.com/environment/2019/oct/05/biosolids-toxic-chemicals-pollution
20 https://www.sas.org.uk
21 https://www.forestresearch.gov.uk/tools-and-resources/fthr/urban-regeneration-and-greenspace-partnership/greenspace-in-practice/planning-integrated-landscapes/sustainable-urban-drainage/
22 SI 1989 No1156, SI 1990 No 1629 and SI 1992 No 339. Scotland has its own Regulations.

References

1 House of Commons Environmental Audit Committee, 2022, *Water quality in rivers Fourth Report of Session 2021–22 report, together with formal minutes relating to the report* https://committees.parliament.uk/publications/8460/documents/88412/default/
2 Bailey SH, 2004, *Garner's Law of Sewers and Drains*, 9th Edition, Shaw and Sons, Kent, UK.

3 National Geographic Education Website, Washington, DC, see https://education. nationalgeographic.org/resource/aquifers/
4 Outdoor Swimming Society Website, see https://www.outdoorswimmingsociety. com/designated-bathing-waters-explained/
5 European Environment Agency, 2021, *French bathing water quality in 2020*, See https://www.eea.europa.eu/en/countries/eea-member-countries/france
6 Defra, 2020, *Report of a review of the arrangements for determining responsibility for surface water and drainage assets*, available at https://assets.publishing. service.gov.uk/government/uploads/system/uploads/attachment_data/file/911812/ surface-water-drainage-review.pdf
7 Giakoumis T and Voulvoulis N, 2023, Combined sewer overflows: relating event duration monitoring data to wastewater systems' capacity in England, *Environmental Science: Water Research & Technology*, Advance Article DOI: 10.1039/ D2EW00637E
8 Professor Chris Whitty, Chief Medical Officer for England, Jonson Cox, Chair, Ofwat, Emma Howard Boyd, Chair, Environment Agency, 2022, *Sewage in water: a growing public health problem*, at https://www.gov.uk/government/news/ sewage-in-water-a-growing-public-health-problem
9 Chislock MF, Doster E, Zitomer RA, and Wilson, AE, 2013, Eutrophication: causes, consequences, and controls in aquatic ecosystems. *Nature Education Knowledge* 4(4):10.
10 Barrett M, Lynch J, and Pond K, undated, *Environmental health impacts on infiltration and exfiltration connected with underground drainage systems*, Report for CROSS (Campaign for the renewal of older sewerage systems), Robens Centre for Public and Environmental Health, University of Surrey, Guildford.
11 Williams B, Clarkson C, Mant C, Drinkwater A, and May E, 2012, Fat, oil and grease deposits in sewers: characterisation of deposits and formation mechanisms, *Water Research*, 46(19):6319–28.
12 Iasmin M, Dean LO, Lappi SE, and Ducoste JJ, 2014, Factors that influence properties of FOG deposits and their formation in sewer collection systems, *Water Research*, 49:92–102.
13 House of Commons Environmental Audit Committee, 2022, Fourth Report of Session 2021–22 "Water Quality in Rivers", HC74.
14 De Benedittis J and Bertrand-Krajewski J-L, 2005, Infiltration in sewer systems: comparison of measurement methods, *Water Science & Technology*, 52(3):219–27.
15 Construction Industry Research and Information Association (CIRIA), 1997, Control of Infiltration to Sewers Report 175, ISBN: 978-0-86017-474-5.
16 Pond K and Bond T, 2022, in Battersby, Ed., *Clay's Handbook of Environmental Health*, Routledge, Abingdon, Oxon.
17 National Infrastructure Commission, 2022, *Reducing the risk of surface water flooding*, London, available at https://nic.org.uk/app/uploads/NIC-Reducing-the-Risk-of-Surface-Water-Flooding-Final-28-Nov-2022.pdf
18 Kimberly-Clark Corporation, 2022, *Forensic evaluation of materials collected at McMillan Pump Station, Jacksonvile, Florida March 12–13 2019*, Jacksonville, FL, available at https://www.kimberly-clark.com/-/media/Kimberly/PDF/safe%20 to%20flush/Legal/JEA%20KCC%20Study%202019.pdf

19 University of Georgia, 2002, Researchers link increased risk of illness to sewage sludge used as fertilizer. *ScienceDaily*. Retrieved April 2, 2023 from www.sciencedaily.com/releases/2002/07/020730075144.htm

20 Local Government Association (LGA) *Sustainable drainage systems*, website at https://www.local.gov.uk/topics/severe-weather/flooding/sustainable-drainage-systems and https://www.susdrain.org, accessed 23 April 2023.

2 Public health and environmental risks from sewage pollution of the environment

In this chapter, the environmental and public health consequences of the discharge of untreated sewage into the aquatic environment are highlighted. It should be noted that sewage that leaks into groundwater (as the result of exfiltration) has the same contents as that discharged via CSO.s and indeed could be at higher concentrations, posing a risk for those working in excavations as well as threats to the environment. The chapter takes account of the implications for environmental and public health, particularly for those who use recreational waters, whether coastal, lakes, or rivers.

As is apparent, even though the sewage is diluted, storm overflows can lead to ecological harm due to their impact on water chemistry. Discharges of raw sewage can contain organic pollutants, microplastics, pharmaceuticals, nutrients, and heavy metals, as well as visible litter from wet wipes and other non-flushable products that are carelessly flushed down toilets. The impact of sewage discharges on ecology varies depending on the pollutants, their concentration, and the nature of the receiving water body. The smaller and more dilute the sewage discharge and the larger and faster flowing the receiving river, in theory at least, the lower should be the ecological impact, but that presumption is questionable given the complex nature of modern sewage. However, with constant and long-standing discharges, some of which have been reported, that presumption becomes somewhat dangerous. For example, one report said the Oxford sewage treatment works have been discharging untreated sewage into the Thames for between 17 and 35 hours a week.[1]

As a 2022 joint press release from the CMO for England and the CEOs of Ofwat and the Environment Agency said "one of the greatest public health triumphs of the last 200 years was separating human faeces from drinking water".[2] It was the basis for preventing cholera, typhoid, and other bacterial and viral diarrhoeal diseases that killed millions in major epidemics. When bacteria from human faeces (coliforms) are ingested, it increases the risk of significant infections, including antibiotic-resistant bacteria. Keeping human faeces out of water people might ingest should be a public health priority.

DOI: 10.1201/9781003375647-2

Threats to human health

Mention has already been made of some of the contents of raw sewage. Here, some of the potential threats to public health as a result of sewage discharge into the environment. This also underlines why this is a public and environmental health issue.

As Brouwer et al. [1] have pointed out, although the waterborne disease burden in high-income countries (HICs) is lower than in low- and middle-income countries (LMICs), outbreaks caused by emerging pathogens and ageing infrastructure have resulted in an increase in research and public health concerns. In both LMICs and HICs, global heating and the resulting changes in temperature, rainfall, and extreme weather have increased the burden of waterborne disease. Sewage can contain waterborne enteric pathogens, including bacteria, viruses, and protozoa, which can exploit a variety of transmission pathways. The major pathogens of concern are strains of *Escherichia coli*, *Salmonella spp.*, *Shigella spp.*, *Campylobacter spp.*, *Vibrio cholerae*, *Cryptosporidium spp.*, *Giardia spp.*, rotavirus, norovirus, poliovirus, and hepatitis A. These pathogens are transmitted through multiple pathways, including water (drinking or recreational water) as well as other pathways [1].

The Indiana Department of Health[3] has listed Campylobacteriosis, Cryptosporidiosis, *E. Coli* diarrhoea, Encephalitis, Gastroenteritis, Giardiasis, Hepatitis A, Leptospirosis, Methaemoglobinaemia, Poliomyelitis, Salmonellosis, Shigellosis, Paratyphoid Fever, Typhoid Fever, and Yersiniosis as diseases caused by sewage or sewage-contaminated water that can occur in the United States. Whether the situation is the same in the UK is unclear, although there is likely to be some commonality.

Campylobacter spp., according to the WHO Campylobacter is one of four key global causes of diarrhoeal diseases. It is considered to be the most common bacterial cause of human gastroenteritis in the world. The main route of transmission is generally believed to be foodborne, via undercooked meat and meat products, as well as raw or contaminated milk. Contaminated water or ice is also a source of infection. A proportion of cases occur following contact with contaminated water during recreational activities.[4] *Campylobacter spp.* Can regularly be found in wastewater-affected surface waters. The occurrence in rivers, treated sewage, and combined sewer overflows was analysed in one study. The highest *Campylobacter spp.* loads and the highest risk of infection were found to occur during the summertime after heavy rainfall [2].

Cryptosporidium spp. is a protozoan parasite that causes a severe diarrhoeal disease known as cryptosporidiosis. Discharge of untreated wastewater may result in waterborne or foodborne outbreaks, but suitable treatment can prevent their dissemination; discharge of raw sewage will not. Most studies on the prevalence of Cryptosporidium oocysts in wastewater have reported a concentration range between 10 and 200 oocysts/L and a prevalence of

6–100%. Activated sludge has been found to be ineffective for the removal of Cryptosporidium oocysts [3].

Nasser [3] concluded that stabilisation ponds and constructed wetlands are efficient for the reduction of *Cryptosporidium* from wastewater, especially when the retention time is longer than 20 days at suitable sunlight and temperature. High-rate filtration and chlorine disinfection, however, are inefficient for the reduction of Cryptosporidium from effluents, whereas ultrafiltration and UV irradiation were found to be very efficient for the reduction of *Cryptosporidium* oocysts.

E. coli and other faecal coliforms: most types of *E. coli* are generally seen as relatively harmless, but they can cause brief diarrhoea. A few strains, however, such as *E. coli* O157:H7, can cause severe stomach cramps, bloody diarrhoea, and vomiting. Healthy adults usually recover from infections with *E. coli* O157:H7 within a week. Young children and older adults have a greater risk of developing a life-threatening form of kidney failure.

As the CMO for England has said, "When bacteria from human faeces (coliforms) are ingested, it increases the risk of significant infections, including antibiotic resistant bacteria. Keeping human faeces out of water people might ingest should be a public health priority".[5]

Coliforms from the continuous normal discharge from sewage works remain a problem as viable bacteria and viruses are discharged as part of normal operations. Eliminating discharges of coliforms from sewage works upstream of popular recreational areas will contribute to reducing human faecal infective organisms downstream. This can be achieved by using ultraviolet treatment.

While much of the focus on health risks has been on people swimming in sewage-polluted waters, it should not be forgotten that shellfish such as oysters, cockles, and mussels will also be contaminated by *E. coli* and other bacteria, leading to the ill-health of consumers.

Giardia spp.: This is another protozoan parasite, and infection is marked by stomach cramps, bloating, nausea, and bouts of watery diarrhoea. Giardia infections are found worldwide, especially in areas with poor sanitation and unsafe water. It can be found in water contaminated by sewage. Giardia infection (giardiasis) is said to be one of the most common causes of waterborne disease in the United States.

Hepatitis: Hepatitis A virus (HAV) is an enteric picornavirus that causes acute hepatitis in humans. It is highly resistant in the environment and typically transmitted via the faecal-oral route through exposure to contaminated foods (raw shellfish, strawberries, etc.) or water, so sewage-polluted water used for recreation is a possible source. However, workers with raw sewage are probably more at risk [4].

In a study in Italy, a total of 38/157 wastewater samples (24.2%) were positive for HAV, 16 collected in 2012 and 22 in 2013. Several HAV strains were detected [5]. These included a variant implicated in an outbreak and isolated from clinical cases over the same period. Italy, like the UK, is a country with low/intermediate endemicity.

Polio: the UK Heath Security Agency (UKHSA) found poliovirus in sewage samples collected from the London Beckton Sewage Treatment Works in 2022.[6] Apparently, it is normal for one to three 'vaccine-like' polioviruses to be detected each year in UK sewage samples, but these have always been one-off findings that were not detected again. These previous detections occurred when an individual vaccinated overseas with the live oral polio vaccine returned or travelled to the UK and briefly 'shed' traces of the vaccine-like poliovirus in their faeces.

Several closely related viruses were found in sewage samples taken between February and May. The virus has continued to evolve and is now classified as a 'vaccine-derived' poliovirus type 2 (VDPV2), which on rare occasions can cause serious illness, such as paralysis, in people who are not fully vaccinated. According to the UKHSA, the detection of a VDPV2 suggests it is likely there has been some spread between closely linked individuals in North and East London and that they are now shedding the type 2 poliovirus strain in their faeces. The last case of wild polio contracted in the UK was confirmed in 1984. The UK was declared polio-free in 2003.

Poliomyelitis (polio) is a highly infectious viral disease that largely affects children under five years of age. The virus is transmitted person-to-person, mainly through the faecal-oral route or, less frequently, by a common vehicle (e.g. contaminated water or food), and multiplies in the intestine, from where it can invade the nervous system and cause paralysis.

The World Health Assembly adopted a resolution in 1988 for the worldwide eradication of polio. Wild poliovirus cases have decreased by over 99% since 1988. Of the three strains of wild poliovirus (types 1–3), wild poliovirus type 2 was eradicated in 1999, and wild poliovirus type 3 was eradicated in 2020. As of 2022, endemic wild poliovirus type 1 remains in two countries, Pakistan and Afghanistan.[7]

The disease may be diagnosed by finding the virus in the faeces or detecting antibodies in the blood.

Salmonella spp.

There are more than 2,500 strains of *Salmonella* bacteria. These live in the guts of domestic and wild animals. Salmonella causes food poisoning. Foods such as eggs, chicken, pork, and dairy products can carry salmonella. Fruit and vegetables can also become contaminated if they have been in contact with livestock, manure, or untreated water. Symptoms of diarrhoea, stomach cramps, nausea, vomiting, and fever usually develop between 12 and 72 hours after becoming infected. The illness usually lasts from four to seven days.

Studies have found the inefficiency of wastewater treatment to remove *Salmonella*, especially since wastewater is considered a good tank for a high diversity of Salmonella serotypes. The identified Salmonella serotypes in the receiving marine environment almost coincide with those identified in wastewater [6]. Salmonella has been isolated from sewage sludge [7] and has been traced back to cases. Although it is said that human gut phages[8] do not seem to replicate during their transit through the sewers, they predominate at the entrance of wastewater treatment plants, inside which the dominant populations of bacteria and phages undergo a swift change. There is growing concern about their potential role in the horizontal transfer of genes, including those related to bacterial pathogenicity and antibiotic resistance [8].

Salmonella enterica is a major cause of gastroenteritis, usually caused by animal-based contaminated foods. Research has found that sewage influent contains Salmonella isolates from humans and that some originated from unreported human cases infected by poultry-associated products [9].

Shigella spp.

Shigella spp. causes shigellosis (bacillary dysentery), and *Shigella* can spread easily from one person to another – and it only takes a small amount of the bacterium to cause illness. Swallowing recreational water contaminated with the bacterium (for example, lake or river water) while swimming can cause the illness.

Shigella can be classified into four major serological groups.[9] Group A, *S. dysenteriae* Group B, *S. flexneri*; Group C, *S. boydii*; and Group D, *S. sonnei*. The last accounts for most cases of dysentery in the developed world. Waterborne outbreaks have generally resulted from inadequate treatment of water or sewage.

S. boydii and *S. dysenteriae* are not indigenous to the UK and occur as travel-associated cases. *S. sonnei* and *S. flexneri* are endemic in the UK, although they can also be travel associated. Primarily a disease of children, over the past ten years in England and Wales, non-travel-associated cases in adults aged 16–60-year old have risen [10].

Vibrio cholerae

Cholera is an acute diarrhoeal infection caused by the ingestion of food or water contaminated with the bacterium *Vibrio cholerae*. Cholera remains a global threat to public health and an indicator of inequity and a lack of social development.

The WHO says it has a short incubation period, ranging between two hours and five days. Most people will develop no or only mild symptoms; less than 20% of ill people develop acute watery diarrhoea with moderate or severe dehydration and are at risk for rapid loss of body fluids, dehydration, and death [11].

Most people infected with *V. cholerae* apparently do not develop any symptoms, although the bacteria are present in their faeces for 1–10 days after infection and are shed back into the environment, potentially infecting other people. For people who develop symptoms, the majority have mild or moderate symptoms, while a minority develop acute watery diarrhoea with severe dehydration. This can lead to death if left untreated.

It is unlikely to be an issue as a result of sewage pollution in the UK because transmission is closely linked to inadequate access to clean water and sanitation facilities. Typical at-risk areas include peri-urban slums and camps for internally displaced persons or refugees, where the minimum requirements of clean water and sanitation are not met. Nevertheless, however slight the risks, there is no room for complacency with global travel or a failure to treat sewage fully.

Chemicals

A 2017 UNESCO study [12] found that the chemicals' main pathway into the freshwater and marine environment was via the discharges of effluents from municipal wastewater treatment plants. Only 9 out of 118 assessed pharmaceuticals were removed from wastewater during the treatment processes with an efficiency of over 95%, and nearly half of the compounds were removed only partially with an efficiency of less than 50%.[10]

Reference has been made to "forever chemicals" in Chapter 1 when discussing sewage sludge. The House of Commons Environmental Audit Committee report on river quality referred to "several submissions highlighted the threat that so-called emerging pollutants such as 'forever chemicals' pose to biodiversity and water quality in rivers" [13]. Chemical pollutants present in river waters include per- and polyfluorinated alkyl substances (PFASs), bisphenols, and flame retardants, all of which are known to affect river water quality, freshwater biota, and human health. Currently, there are more than 4,700 different PFAS that accumulate in people and the environment [14]. According to the US EPA [15], current peer-reviewed scientific studies have shown that exposure to certain levels of PFAS may lead to:

- Reproductive effects such as decreased fertility or increased blood pressure in pregnant women
- Developmental effects or delays in children, including low birth weight, accelerated puberty, bone variations, or behavioural changes
- Increased risk of some cancers, including prostate, kidney, and testicular cancers
- Reduced ability of the body's immune system to fight infections, including reduced vaccine response

- Interference with the body's natural hormones
- Increased cholesterol levels and/or risk of obesity

Metals

Sewage pollution can result in increasing levels of trace elements in the environment. One study looked at the role of sewage discharges in the contamination of aquatic systems, especially on rocky shores where food resources are collected from coastal waters. For this purpose, the accumulation of trace elements (Copper, Zinc, Lead, Nickel, Cobalt, Cadmium, Iron, Manganese, and Arsenic) by edible molluscs was compared between one sewage-impacted area and two reference areas. This study suggested that the concentrations of trace elements in the soft tissues of the selected molluscs can be affected by the presence of sewage discharges. The sewage pollution increased the concentrations of arsenic in the mollusc species, which highlighted the potential damaging effects on natural systems, edible species, and human health where such molluscs are consumed [16].

Antibiotics and other pharmaceuticals

There is concern regarding environmental contamination with pharmaceuticals, with the European Commission[11] recognising that pollution of waters and soils with pharmaceuticals is an emerging environmental issue and also a critical concern for public health [17]. Humans can subsequently be exposed through drinking water and ingestion of pharmaceutical residues in plant crops, fish, dairy products, and meat [18].

The presence of antibiotics in the aquatic environment is a serious concern because of concerns that it may accelerate the proliferation of antibiotic-resistant pathogens through genetic mutations and resistance vectors with a high transfer rate between pathogens. This will lower the therapeutic effect of antibiotics. In addition, it is said that antimicrobial resistance can be transferred between different organisms throughout the food chain. According to the World Health Organization, antimicrobial resistance is a significant challenge to global human and animal health and food safety [19].

Improper disposal of antibiotics, for example, by households that flush antibiotics down the toilet, could represent a significant factor in the antibiotic's occurrence in wastewater systems. A lack of proper medication disposal practices among patients and clinicians requires targeted information about the effects of improper disposal on the environment. It has been found that the contribution of the release of antibiotics into the environment to the spread and maintenance of clinically relevant antibiotic resistance is correlated with antibiotic consumption patterns [20].

Human pharmaceuticals and their metabolites affect the endocrine system and physiology of aquatic wildlife, which is an important global ecological concern. Published data from open-source toxicology and worldwide web resources reveal about 175 pharmaceuticals that can affect oestrogen pathways to disrupt the endocrine system and metabolism [21].

The presence of nine hormones and their conjugates and pharmaceuticals such as anti-inflammatories, lipid regulators, and antibiotics, among others, has been found in sewage sludge from sewage treatment plants, indicating what will be contained in untreated sewage. It has been argued that their unknown toxicity, teratogenicity, and carcinogenicity profiles associated with a lack of monitoring and control measures impose a significant hazard risk on the public health [22].

Some studies have indicated that pharmaceuticals, e.g., carbamazepine, diclofenac, and gabapentin, artificial sweeteners, e.g., acesulfame, X-ray contrast media (e.g., iohexol and iopromide), and corrosion inhibitors (e.g., benzotriazole, which is also a UV stabiliser and is an emerging contaminant widely used in personal care products, such as cosmetics and sunscreens, to absorb ultraviolet light [23]) are only partially removed in conventional wastewater treatment processes. The risks to human health do not appear to have been assessed. As has been cautioned for carbamazepine and diclofenac, the ecotoxicological studies of both drugs imply that they do not easily cause acute toxic effects at their environmental concentrations. "However, their chronic effects need cautious attention" [24].

Microplastics

The term is used to differentiate microplastics from larger plastic waste, such as plastic bottles. Two classifications of microplastics are currently recognised. Primary microplastics include any plastic fragments or particles that are 5.0 mm in size or less before entering the environment. These include microfibres from clothing microbeads and plastic pellets (also known as nurdles). Secondary microplastics arise from the degradation (breakdown) of larger plastic products through natural weathering processes after entering the environment. Such sources of secondary microplastics include water and soda bottles, fishing nets, plastic bags, microwave containers, tea bags, and vehicle tyre wear.

Marine plastic waste pollution is considered to be one of the greatest and most urgent marine environmental problems. Research has reviewed the current state of knowledge and shown that plastic waste is not biodegradable and can only be broken down, predominantly by physical processes, into small particles of micron to nanometre size. Particles (<150 μm) can be ingested by living organisms, migrate through the intestinal wall, and reach lymph nodes and other organs. The primary pathways of human exposure to micro-plastics have been identified as gastrointestinal ingestion via sea food, pulmonary inhalation, and dermal infiltration. They may pollute drinking water, accumulate in the food chain, and release toxic chemicals that may cause disease, including certain cancers. Micro/nanoplastics may pose acute toxicity, (sub) chronic toxicity, carcinogenicity, genotoxicity, and developmental toxicity. In addition, nanoplastics may pose chronic toxicity (cardiovascular toxicity, hepatotoxicity, and neurotoxicity [25]. Again, there are many unknowns when it comes to the evaluation of risks for the marine ecosystem and human health as a result of microplastics and nanoplastics.

Threats to the environment and aquatic ecosystem

Although separated out here, in reality, threats to the environment or ecosystem end up being threats to human health, as we have seen above. For example, algal blooms are encouraged by the presence of sewage and can lead to the deaths of other species, a negative change in biodiversity, and an impact on the functioning of an ecosystem. Such blooms can change a whole river. While the focus of this work is on the impact of sewage discharges, agricultural run-off can add to the increased risk of algal blooms.

Sewage contains substantial amounts of nitrogen and phosphorous, which are nutrients. These stimulate the growth of algae and biofilms in sediments, leading to algal blooms, which, in turn, remove oxygen from the water. Algae also block out the light that plants need for photosynthesis. When these plants and the algae start to die, they are then consumed by bacteria, which reduces oxygen in the water, killing fish and other organisms. Freshwater insects are badly affected by a lack of oxygen, many of which spend large periods of their development in rivers. Eutrophication of bodies of water is characterised by excessive plant and algal growth.

Algal blooms and eutrophication lead to an increased Biological Chemical Demand (BOD), which can lead to a change in biodiversity with fish dying off. The whole character of a river system can thus be changed.

Poor water quality creates conditions for a small minority of plants and organisms to thrive and others to suffer further sustained loss in both abundance and diversity. This affects invertebrates, plants, and animals, as set out in the Troubled Waters Report [26]. This highlights that in England, only 14% of rivers meet standards for good ecological status, with less than half achieving these standards in Wales. In Northern Ireland, only 31% of water bodies are classified as good or high quality. "The poor health of many of our waterways has a significant impact on nature, with many species in decline and some facing extinction". While sewage pollution is not the sole cause, agricultural run-off, which includes excess nutrients as well as pesticides and herbicides, is a major contributory factor to the poor ecological quality of rivers and coastal waters.

Notes

1 See: https://www.theguardian.com/environment/2023/jan/11/thames-water-criticised-lack-investment-sewage-treatment-works; https://www.theguardian.com/environment/2023/jan/23/thames-waters-real-time-map-raw-sewage-discharges-rivers; and https://www.walesonline.co.uk/news/wales-news/every-place-raw-sewage-dumped-23118117
2 https://www.gov.uk/government/news/sewage-in-water-a-growing-public-health-problem
3 See: https://www.in.gov/health/eph/onsite-sewage-systems-program/diseases-involving-sewage/
4 See: https://www.who.int/news-room/fact-sheets/detail/campylobacter
5 Ibid., p1.
6 See: https://www.gov.uk/government/news/poliovirus-detected-in-sewage-from-north-and-east-london
7 See: https://www.who.int/health-topics/poliomyelitis/#tab=tab_1
8 These are viruses that solely kill and selectively target bacteria.
9 https://www.sciencedirect.com/topics/immunology-and-microbiology/shigella
10 See: https://www.unep.org/news-and-stories/story/drugged-waters-how-modern-medicine-turning-environmental-curse
11 See: https://health.ec.europa.eu/medicinal-products/pharmaceuticals-and-environment_en

References

1 Brouwer AF, Masters NB, and Eisenberg JNS, 2018 Jun, Quantitative microbial risk assessment and infectious disease transmission modelling of waterborne enteric pathogens. *Current Environmental Health Reports*, 5(2):293–304. DOI: 10.1007/s40572-018-0196-x. PMID: 29679300; PMCID: PMC5984175
2 Rechenburg A and Kistemann T, 2009 Aug, Sewage effluent as a source of Campylobacter sp. in a surface water catchment. *International Journal of Environmental Health Research*, 19(4):239–49. DOI: 10.1080/09603120802460376. PMID: 20183194.
3 Abidelfatah M Nasser, 2016 Feb, Removal of Cryptosporidium by wastewater treatment processes: a review. *Journal of Water and Health*, 14(1):1–13. DOI: 10.2166/wh.2015.131
4 Brugha R, Heptonstall J, Farrington P, Andren S, Perry K, and Parry J, 1998 Aug, Risk of hepatitis A infection in sewage workers. *Occupational and Environmental Medicine*, 55(8):567–69. DOI: 10.1136/oem.55.8.567. PMID: 9849545; PMCID: PMC1757623.
5 La Rosa et al., 2014, Surveillance of hepatitis A virus in urban sewages and comparison with cases notified in the course of an outbreak, Italy 2013, *BMC Infectious Diseases*, 14:419 at http://www.biomedcentral.com/1471-2334/14/419
6 El Boulani A and Mimouni R et al., 2017, Salmonella in wastewater: Identification, antibiotic resistance and the impact on the marine environment, in Mares M., Ed., *Current Topics in Salmonella and Salmonellosis* [Internet]. InTech. Available from: http://dx.doi.org/10.5772/63008
7 Sahlström L, de Jong B, and Aspan A, 2006 Jul, Salmonella isolated in sewage sludge traced back to human cases of salmonellosis. *Letters in Applied Microbiology*, 43(1):46–52. DOI: 10.1111/j.1472-765X.2006.01911.x. PMID: 16834720.

8 Ballesté E, Blanch AR, and Muniesa M et al., 2022, Bacteriophages in sewage: abundance, roles, and applications, *FEMS Microbes*, 3, xtac009, https://doi.org/10.1093/femsmc/xtac009

9 Yanagimoto K and Yamagami T et al., 2020 Jan, Characterization of *Salmonella* isolates from wastewater treatment plant influents to estimate unreported cases and infection sources of Salmonellosis. *Pathogens*, 9(1):52. DOI: 10.3390/pathogens9010052. PMID: 31936747; PMCID: PMC7168602.

10 Public Health England Website (updated 4 January 2019) see: https://www.gov.uk/government/collections/shigella-guidance-data-and-analysis, accessed 23 April 2023.

11 WHO, *Cholera - Global situation*, website https://www.who.int/emergencies/disease-outbreak-news/item/2022-DON426, accessed 23 April 2023.

12 UNESCO, 2017, *Pharmaceuticals in the aquatic environment of the Baltic Sea region: a status report*, Emerging Pollutants in Water Series, The United Nations Educational, Scientific and Cultural Organization, Paris, at https://www.helcom.fi/wp-content/uploads/2019/08/BSEP149.pdf

13 House of Commons Environmental Audit Committee, 2022, Fourth Report of Session 2021–22 "Water Quality in Rivers", HC74.

14 European Environment Agency Website Infographic - *Effects of PFAS on human health*, at https://www.eea.europa.eu/signals/signals-2020/infographics/effects-of-pfas-on-human-health/view, accessed 23 April 2023.

15 US EPA, Website Our *Current understanding of the human health and environmental risks of PFAS*, https://www.epa.gov/pfas/our-current-understanding-human-health-and-environmental-risks-pfas.

16 Cabral-Oliveira J and Pratas J et al., 2015, Trace elements in edible rocky shore species: effect of sewage discharges and human health risk implications, *Human and Ecological Risk Assessment: An International Journal*, 21(1):135–45, DOI: 10.1080/10807039.2014.890480

17 European Commission, 2019, Communication from the Commission, European Union Strategic Approach to Pharmaceuticals in the Environment COM(2019) 128 final.

18 OECD, 2019, *Pharmaceutical residues in freshwater: hazards and policy responses*, OECD Studies on Water, OECD Publishing, Paris.

19 Sosa-Hernández JE et al., 2021 Dec, Sources of antibiotics pollutants in the aquatic environment under SARS-CoV-2 pandemic situation, *Case Studies in Chemical and Environmental Engineering*, 4:100127, https://doi.org/10.1016/j.cscee.2021.100127.

20 Polianciuc SJ et al., 2020, Antibiotics in the environment: causes and consequences, *Medicine and Pharmacy Reports,* 93(3):231–40.

21 Srivastava B and Reddy PB, 2021, Impacts of human pharmaceuticals on fish health, *International Journal of Pharmaceutical Sciences and Research*, DOI: 10.13040/IJPSR.0975-8232.12(10).5185-94 at https://ijpsr.com/bft-article/impacts-of-human-pharmaceuticals-on-fish-health/

22 Nassiri Koopaei N and Abdollahi M, 2017 Apr, Health risks associated with the pharmaceuticals in wastewater. *DARU Journal of Pharmaceutical Sciences*, 25(1):9. DOI: 10.1186/s40199-017-0176-y. PMID: 28403898; PMCID: PMC5389172

23 Montesdeoca-Esponda S and Álvarez-Raya C et al., 2019 Mar, Monitoring and environmental risk assessment of benzotriazole UV stabilizers in the sewage and coastal environment of Gran Canaria (Canary Islands, Spain). *Journal of Environmental Management*, 233:567–75.

24 Zhang Y, Geissen SU, and Gal C, 2008 Nov, Carbamazepine and diclofenac: removal in wastewater treatment plants and occurrence in water bodies. *Chemosphere*. 73(8):1151–61. DOI: 10.1016/j.chemosphere.2008.07.086. Epub 2008 Sep 14. PMID: 18793791.

25 Yuan Z, Nag R, and Cummins E, 2022, Human health concerns regarding microplastics in the aquatic environment - From marine to food systems, *Science of the Total Environment*, 823:153730.

26 RSPB, 2021, *Troubled Waters* at https://www.rspb.org.uk/about-the-rspb/about-us/media-centre/press-releases/troubled-waters-report/ (report from RSPB, The Wildlife Trusts, Rivers Trust, National Trust, Afonydd Cymru and Wales Environment Link).

3   The legal framework and cases

This chapter will examine the law as it affects sewerage from our homes and buildings to the wider environment. The first section will look at legislation specifically relating to the water and sewerage industry, including privatisation of the water and sewerage industry in England and Wales, and its impact is also relevant. It should not be forgotten that these private companies fulfil an essential public health function, and private water companies are public authorities for the purposes of the Environmental Information Regulations 2004 (EIR) and the Environmental Information (Scotland) Regulations 2004 (EIR-S).[1]

The law on how sewers and lateral drains become the responsibility of the WaSCs will be examined, as well as provisions on connecting drainage to these sewers. There will also be reference to any changes introduced by the Environment Act 2021 on storm overflows. In addition to controls on polluting discharges from sewage treatment works, this section will look at the law on discharges to sewers.

The second part of the chapter will focus on the law as it affects near-house drainage and will include misconnections around dwellings. This is an important consideration and an illustration that there cannot be a hard and fast demarcation between the two sections, as misconnections can lead to pollution of water bodies.

The chapter will finally examine leading cases on drains, sewers, and sewage pollution.

Privatisation and Water Industry Act 1989

A little context

Prior to 1974, controls over the provision and maintenance of sewers and drains were almost solely the responsibility of local authorities, with some central government supervision. There is a line from the Public Health Acts of 1848 and 1875 to that of 1936, with minor amendments in the 1961 Act. In Scotland, the Sewerage (Scotland) Act 1968 (as amended) says "Subject

DOI: 10.1201/9781003375647-3

to the provisions of this Act, it shall be the duty of Scottish Water[2] to provide such public sewers and public sustainable drainage systems (SuDs) systems (see later on SuDS) as may be necessary". In Northern Ireland, NI Water, which formerly was an executive agency within the Northern Ireland Executive, became a government-owned company in April 2007 and now sits as an Agency within the Department of Infrastructure. NI Water has responsibility for sewerage and water supply.

In England and Wales, the Water Act 1973 transferred many of the functions that had been the responsibility of local authorities to the ten regional water authorities (RWAs) in England and Wales, and the public sewers of the local authorities were then vested in these new authorities. These water authorities were then privatised by the Water Act 1989; we then had the Water Industry Act 1991 (WIA'91), and these became Water and Sewerage Companies (WaSCs).

Privatisation and implications

Privatisation was originally proposed in 1984 and again in 1986, but there was strong public objection to the proposals. However, after the election of 1987, the privatisation plan was resurrected and implemented. Water privatisation in England involved the transfer of the provision of water and wastewater services from the RWAs in the public sector to the private sector in 1989. The ten regional RWAs were then sold, and the private water-only companies (the statutory water companies) remained in the private sector. The RWAs supplied both the public water supply as well as the sewerage and sewage disposal functions; these services were transferred to privately owned companies (Water and Sewerage Companies (WSCs)).

The WSCs paid £7.6 billion for the RWAs. At the same time, the government assumed responsibility for the sector's total debts amounting to £5 billion and granted the WSCs a further £1.5 billion of public funds.[3]

England and Wales are the only countries in the world to have a fully privatised water and sewage disposal system. Since 2001, in Wales, Welsh Water (Dwr Cymru) has operated as a single-purpose, not-for-profit company with no shareholders, "run solely for the benefit of customers". In Scotland and Northern Ireland, water and sewerage services are provided by government entities and not privatised. According to *The Guardian* newspaper, the English WSCs are now mostly owned by foreign investment firms, private equity, pension funds, and businesses lodged in tax havens, so tax avoidance strategies are in place. In total, they own more than 70% of the water industry.[4]

It is questionable whether water privatisation was ever really about efficiency or investment. In the short term, it seems the overriding political priority was a "successful" sale (even if the water industry was never a truly "nationalised" industry). It so happened that the view was that demand for shares was high, and it was important that those who had applied and, from previous privatisations, had come to expect a large premium, were not disappointed.

Thus, as was argued in the *Financial Times*, the Treasury's position was weak when seeking a higher share price or tighter regulation to limit bills in the future, and regrettably, tighter regulation never seems to have been an option. The National Audit Office report on the sale detailed how the forecast proceeds fell by more than a third over just three months, costing taxpayers as Camilla Cavendish wrote in the *Financial Times* [1].

It has also been reported in the Financial Times (FT) that English water companies leak about 20% of their water supply, compared with 5–7% in Germany. It was reported that water companies lost an average of 2,923.8 m litres of water a day in 2021–22, equating to 1.06 tn litres over the year.[5] In some cases, this water can pass into the sewer through infiltration where there are defects, e.g., poor joints and cracks, thereby increasing the flow and reducing the efficiency of treatment. This is in addition to any groundwater that can infiltrate into the sewers where the water table is high and there are defects.

It seems now to be routine for there to be discharges of raw sewage into rivers and on to beaches, which then harm bathing water quality as well as pose risks to public health, as we have seen earlier in the book. In 2021, Southern Water pleaded guilty to knowingly permitting noxious matter to enter rivers and seas when the Environment Agency (EA) brought a prosecution alleging 51 offences caused by deliberate failings at 16 wastewater treatment works and one storm overflow. SWS admitted to causing 6,971 illegal discharges over the offending period (2010–105), which lasted a total of 61,704 hours, the equivalent of 2,571 days or just over seven years. Running its treatment plans below capacity, it had dumped raw sewage into protected seas, contaminating shellfish and acting as the judge said,[6]

> each of the 51 offences seen in isolation shows a shocking and wholesale disregard for the environment, for the precious and delicate ecosystems along the North Kent and Solent coastlines, for human health, and for the fisheries and other legitimate businesses that depend on the vitality of the coastal waters.

The government seems to consider that high levels of self-reporting demonstrate transparency and honesty, yet for the period 2015–2020, what the government considered "high-level" was at least "75% of incidents self-reported by 2020".[7] The thinking is that without it, public agencies would "be reliant on third parties to report when things have gone wrong" – yet what are the regulators for, and in any event, it is the "public and third parties" that have highlighted the issue? The Environment Agency suggests companies report only 77% of incidents, which is not what might be expected at a "high level". Even the Chair of the Environment Agency said the "sector performance for serious pollution incident numbers was much worse than 2020, and there has been no sustained trend for improvement for several years in total incident numbers or compliance with conditions for discharging treated wastewater". It is only thanks to third parties, including the musician Feargal Sharkey, Surfers Against Sewage, and independent scientists who have taken samples, that the scale of the problem has been exposed.

It was argued in 1989 that privatisation would lead to greater efficiency and investment. That does not appear to be true in practice, as the Southern Water case illustrates. The FT's analysis suggests that water companies have cut investment in critical infrastructure by a fifth since the 1990s. It was reported in 1998[8] in a report for the Department for Environment Transport, and Regional Affairs Select Committee that Since 1991, 1,200 km of sewers had been renovated, and this implied a renewal rate of less than 1%. Capital expenditure on sewerage in the period was about £3 billion. Estimates in that report varied for how long sewers would have to last in theory if this rate of renewal was not improved. The highest figure was a thousand years; other estimates were 500 and 400 years. It was further estimated that it would take "almost forty years" to replace the poorest sewers (8–10% of the total network), even assuming that there was no deterioration in the majority. This report was from 25 years ago, but there is no evidence that the rate of renewal has improved.

According to David Hall (Visiting Professor, Public Services International Research Unit (PSIRU)),

The promise of privatisation was that private shareholders would make the investments needed, but the reverse has happened. In 2019, the English companies had a total of £14.7 billion in shareholder equity on their balance sheets, less in value than the money they had put into the companies in 1991. In reality, investments have been entirely financed from customer payments [2].

The evidence from Scotland shows that public ownership, by contrast, can deliver more investment at a lower cost to consumers [3]. "Scottish Water invested nearly 35% more per household since 2002 (average £282 per household per year vs England's £210 per year). Had the English companies invested at that rate, £28 billion more could have gone into the infrastructure" [3].

Water Industry Act 1991 (WIA'91)

This Act has been amended by a number of subsequent Acts, and this is mentioned as issues are discussed.

Provision of public sewers and requisition

Section 94 of the WIA'91 places duty on the sewerage undertaker to

provide, improve and extend such as system of public sewers (whether inside is area or elsewhere)............. and so to cleanse and maintain those sewers and any lateral drains as to ensure that that area is and continually to be effectually drained;.

This is similar to what was the Water Act 1973 and previously s.14 of the Public Health Act 1936, and before that, s.15 of the Public Health Act 1875.

This duty is enforceable by s.18 by the Secretary of State or, with the Secretary of State's authorisation or consent, the Water Services Regulation Authority via an 'enforcement order'. Contravention of an enforcement order is actionable by a person affected or who suffers loss or damage. In *Dear v Thames Water* (1993) 33 Con.L.R. 43, it was held that an action against the sewerage undertaker in respect of alleged negligence or nuisance occurring after 31 August 1989 in respect of matters coming within the enforcement procedure was precluded. See also *Marcic v Thames Water* later. There is a due diligence defence.

Sections 23 & 24 of the 1991 Act provide for the issue of special administration orders by the High Court in certain cases of default.

Section 98 of WIA'91 provides that a sewerage undertaker is under a duty to provide a public sewer or public lateral drain for the drainage of domestic purposes where it is required to do so by a notice (a "requisition notice") served on it by one or more persons entitled to make such a demand, owners or occupiers of premises within its area. Local authorities may also serve requisition notices. The sewerage undertaker may impose financial conditions upon those making the requisition, except where the requisition is by the local authority. The sewerage undertaker may require from those requisitioning a sewer undertakings that they will pay over the 12 years following the provision of the sewer the 'relevant deficit' – the difference between the sewerage charge and the borrowing costs of a loan required to provide the sewer where the latter exceeds the former.

Section 101A (introduced by the Environment Act 1995) introduced an obligation to provide a public sewer for the drainage of domestic premises in certain circumstances:

i Premises to be drained were erected or substantially completed by 20 June 1995 (Date now removed by the Water Act 2003)
ii The drains or sewers used for the drainage of domestic sewerage do not connect with a public sewer
iii The existing drainage is giving rise, or is likely to give rise, to such adverse environmental or amenity effects that it is appropriate (having regard to the Secretary of State's guidance) and all other relevant considerations such as the geology, number of premises, costs of providing the sewer, nature and extent of adverse effects, and the extent to which it is practicable for those effects to be overcome by the provisions of a public sewer.

In brief, the provision of public sewerage in areas hitherto unserved in that way.

The sewerage undertaker carries out an economic and technical appraisal before deciding whether a sewer is the most cost-effective solution, and the criteria for assessment can be summarised as:

- There is a risk to water sources
- There is evidence of a risk to public health from the existing system, but not neglect
- Polluting matter is reaching or can reach a watercourse
- Sewage pollution is damaging the local amenity value
- There are breaches of other statutory requirements resulting in environmental problems
- Other practical technical issues that need to be considered
- Costs of the proposed sewer and any alternatives

The Environment Agency is responsible for making decisions on any disputes. The power to charge for services under s.101A is to be exercised through a charging scheme applicable to the undertaker's customers generally, but see *R (on application of Anglian Water Services Ltd) v Environment Agency* [2000] EWHC, N.P.C 113[9] on how the Agency should reach a decision in this matter.

In *R (on the application of Dwr Cymru (Welsh Water)) v Environment Agency* [2009] EWHC 453 (Admin) [2009] 11 EG 118 (CS), there was a dispute as to the timing of the provision of a public sewer under s.101A. The claimant had originally accepted the duty but changed its mind and notified the local authority. Complaints had been made by residents as far back as 1998. The local authority referred the dispute to the EA, which had ordered that a public sewer be provided by March 2010. The claim for judicial review was dismissed. The claimant had established no legal basis on which it was entitled to withdraw or revoke a 2005 decision to the effect that a duty to provide a sewer existed. The judgement also contains general observations concerning cost-benefit assessment in the environmental field and the procedure in disputes referred to the Environment Agency under Section 101A(7).

Once it is established that a line of pipes carrying effluent from buildings is a sewer rather than a drain (in general, s.101A is not applicable where problems relate to only one building), and when defects have been identified, then s.101A will be applicable. It is worth noting that public sewers as has been noted above, are those vested in the sewerage undertaker, but this may be the result of sewers having been vested in a local authority many years previously, long before any local government reorganisation.

A newly constructed sewer will be a public sewer and vested in the sewerage undertaker if it is laid by the undertaker; the sewerage undertaker has made a declaration of vesting (adopted it); or it is laid in the undertaker's area under the Highways Act 1980 (making up of private streets to be public highways) and is not a sewer belonging to a road maintained by the highway authority.

Adoption

WaSCs can adopt sewers where they have not built and provided the pipeline themselves. Under s.102 of the WIA'91, the WaSC may adopt by declaration any sewer or lateral drain that connects with a public sewer, which then becomes vested in the WaSC. An owner of such an existing sewer or lateral drain can apply for it to be adopted. Under s.104, the WaSC and anyone building a sewer or lateral may enter into an agreement that, when built, it will be adopted.

The Guidance on Design and Construction [3] is for use by developers when planning, designing, and constructing foul and surface water drainage systems (including pumping stations and rising mains) intended for adoption under an agreement made in accordance with Section 104. The latest version was published in June 2022 [4]. There are also model agreements for use under s.104, discussed further below. Ofwat has prepared Sector Guidance in relation to the adoption of sewerage assets by sewerage companies in England; the latest version also being published in June 2022. This contains a draft Model Sewerage Adoption Agreement and can be found on the Water UK website.[10]

An adoption agreement by a WaSC with a developer is one way the developer can demonstrate to a local planning authority that provision has been made for the future maintenance of the drainage system. The sewerage undertaker may at any time adopt any sewer or part of a sewer provided the appropriate procedure is followed and the construction was not completed before 1 October 1937 (see s.102 of the WIA'91). The effect of any declaration of adoption is to cause the sewer to vest in the sewerage undertaker from the date of declaration.

Any person entitled to use the sewer before the declaration shall be able to use the sewer to the same extent after. It is unlikely that a sewerage undertaker would be immune from liability for any damage caused by a former defective private sewer (that is, it was a private sewer before the 2011 Regulations came into force[11]) that had been adopted. However, a sewerage undertaker would probably not be liable for any damage caused by an improperly or negligently constructed sewer that had been vested in it by virtue of statute, e.g., under s.13 of the Public Health Act 1875, or whether with or against their will.

The procedure for adoption (whether or not an owner has made an application under s.102 of the 1991 Act):

- Notice to owners, including owners of easements, must be in writing (see, for example, *Epping Forest DC v Essex Rendering* [1983] 1 All ER 359; [1983] 1 WLR 158; 81 LGR 252; 147 JP 101; 127 Sol Jo 84; even though this case related to an offensive trade offence, it established that consent has to be in writing
- If sewers are outside the area of the undertaker, notice must be given to the undertaker in whose area sewers are located

- No vesting declaration may be made (except on the application of such a body) in respect of any sewer or part thereof that is vested in another sewerage undertaker, a local authority, county council, railway undertaker, or dock undertaker

When notice has been served, the adopting undertaker cannot proceed until either the period of two months has elapsed without an appeal against the proposals or until such an appeal has been determined. The owner of any sewer aggrieved by the proposal may appeal to the Director General within two months of service of the notice. A similar right is available to any owner aggrieved by the refusal of an undertaker to make a vesting declaration.

Under s.102, when a sewerage undertaker considers whether to make a vesting declaration or when Ofwat considers an appeal, regard must be had to all circumstances, and more specifically:

- Whether the sewer in question is adapted to, or required for, any general system of sewerage that the undertaker has provided or proposes to provide
- Whether the sewer is constructed under a highway or under land reserved by a planning scheme for a street (The Secretary of State suggested that adoption should not be refused on this ground merely because sewers are in back gardens, given undertakers' powers of entry and local authority powers to prevent construction over a sewer, *Re Westfield Drive, Bolton le Sands*, DoE Appeal Decision, October 15, 1987, WS/5527/AB/17, although in 2011 guidance Defra has suggested rear gardens should be avoided[12])
- The number of buildings which the sewer is intended to serve, and given the proximity of other buildings and the prospect of future developments, it is likely to be required to serve additional buildings
- The method of construction and state of repair of the sewer
- In a case where an owner objects, whether the making of the proposed vesting declaration would be seriously detrimental to him, e.g., increased likelihood that sewer would overflow onto his land, or that some structural failure could arise

Under s.104 of the WRA'91 (as amended by s.11 of the Water Act 2014), the sewerage undertaker can agree to a request from the person building a sewer, such as on a new housing development, to make an agreement to adopt the sewer so long as it is constructed in accordance with the required standard as set out in Ofwat's *Guidance for foul and surface water sewers offered for adoption under the Code* [3]. Ofwat has decided that generally, sewers should be adopted if:

- The development and associated sewerage have been planned in a way that provides efficient drainage of the properties

• The design and standard of construction comply with the Guidance referred to above. (Nevertheless, it is still possible, at least in theory, for a sewerage undertaker to have their own individual requirements and conditions, for example, on pipe materials)
• There are no outstanding maintenance problems, and the sewers are in satisfactory condition
• The sewers are compatible with the existing sewer system, so no operational problems would arise
• There is easy access for maintenance purposes (i.e. laid in the highway or land open to the public)

Sewer maps

Under Section 199 of the 1991 Act, the sewerage undertakers are required to keep records of the location of every sewer vested in the company. Section 200 of the Act places a duty on sewerage undertakers to provide local authorities with copies of these records and any modifications made to them. They are also required to make sewer records available for public inspection free of charge. A sewerage undertaker, however, is not required to record drains, sewers, or disposal mains laid prior to 1 September 1989 if it has no knowledge of or reasonable grounds to suspect their presence or if it is not reasonably practicable for it to discover their course (s.199(7)). The undertakers were not under a duty from that date and for ten years to record any drain, sewer, or disposal main that was laid before that date unless particulars of it were shown immediately prior to that date on a map kept by the local authority.

It is likely that not all sewers and lateral drains that are now vested in the WaSCs appear on the sewer maps. EHPs will need to treat these maps with caution, and the fact that a sewer does not appear on the map does not mean that it is not the responsibility of the WaSC. This book will hopefully provide some pointers as to the possible status of pipelines and where responsibilities lie.

The 1991 Act was amended by the Water Act 2003 in a number of ways, and these are discussed in the next section. Further amendments to this Act made by subsequent Acts are also discussed in the sections on those Acts.

Water Act 2003

The Water Act 2003 was intended to take on the Government's commitment to the sustainable management and use of water resources. It updated the framework for abstraction licencing, promoted greater water conservation and planning for the future by water companies, and is intended to build a more stable and transparent regulatory environment that puts the consumer at the heart of regulation. It also amended the 1991 Act, and some of those amendments have already been considered.

Sections 93, 94, 95 96, 97, 98, & 99 of the 2003 Act amended the WIA'91, as we have seen, establishing the concept of "public laterals" already discussed and amended provisions for:

- The requisition and adoption of sewers (and the financial arrangements)
- The provision of public sewers other than by requisition
- The requisition of lateral drains means that part of a drain that runs from the curtilage of a building (or buildings or yards within the same curtilage) to the sewer with which the drain communicates or is to communicate
- The adoption of lateral drains (so there are "public lateral drains" – drains that either belong to the sewerage undertaker or are vested in the sewerage undertaker by virtue of a declaration made under Section 102 above or under an agreement made under Section 104 above
- Communication of laterals with public sewers (s.106)

The Act provides that:

- New laterals may not be connected to a public sewer unless they are built to an adoptable standard
- Adoption agreements may require inspection chambers (demarcation chambers) to be constructed to an adoptable standard close to the curtilage of the property to act as a demarcation point between the drain from the property (which remains the householder's responsibility) and the lateral (which becomes the sewerage undertaker's responsibility)

Private sewers and laterals outside the curtilage have now been transferred to the WaSCs, with two exceptions; these are private sewers that only conveyed rainwater to watercourses and some privately owned pumping stations.

Connection to a public sewer

Under s.106 of the WIA'91 (as amended), the owner or occupier of any premises or the owner of a sewer that is not a public sewer is entitled to have the drain or sewer communicate with the public sewer. This right now also extends to connections with public lateral drains. The right is subject to the owner having the right (either by ownership or easement) to have that drain or sewer pass through the intervening land. This does not apply where the liquid is from a factory, other than domestic sewage, surface or storm water, or any liquid from a manufacturing process, or is a liquid or other matter the discharge of which into sewers is prohibited.

Since May 2004, the right to connect to a public sewer or public lateral drain is also subject to the drain or sewer being built to an adoptable standard (already discussed). This will be obvious for new laterals, as there will be a "demarcation chamber" at the curtilage. This would mark the boundary between what could be adopted, making it a public lateral, and what would remain the owner/occupier's responsibility.

To exercise this right, the person seeking to make the connection must give the sewerage undertaker written notice (no prescribed wording), and within 21 days of receipt, the undertaker may by written notice refuse permission for the communication if it appears that the mode of construction or condition of the drain or sewer does not meet the standards required by the undertaker or that making such a connection would prejudice the working of the undertaker's system, e.g., a 12-inch private sewer connecting to a 4-inch public sewer.

However, it would seem not to be reasonable for the undertaker to refuse permission just because the discharge might surcharge the public sewer or otherwise cause a nuisance (see *Smeaton v Ilford Corporation*) [1954] Ch. 450). In that case, it was held that even if the local authority was responsible for the sewage affecting Smeaton, overloading arose not from any act of the defendant corporation but because, under legislation (then Section 34 of the Public Health Act 1936), they were obliged to permit occupiers of premises to make connections to the sewer and to discharge their sewage therein. The fact that a sewer is already overloaded is therefore not necessarily a ground for refusing permission for connection. See also *Barratt Homes Ltd v Dwr Cymru (Welsh Water)* [2008] EWCA Civ 1552. (The WaSC wanted the connection some distance from where the developer wanted it.) Accepting that decision, there was still an appeal to the Supreme Court, and Dwr Cymru was anxious to establish that a sewerage undertaker has a right to refuse to permit a connection to be made to one of their sewers. This is discussed further below. Also see the later section on cases for continuing issues in this saga in *Barratt Homes Ltd v Dwr Cymru* [2013] EWCA Civ 233.

This right of communication for owners or occupiers only applies to sewers or drains as defined in the 1991 Act, and anyone wishing to "avail" themselves of this provision shall give the WaSC notice. Any person making a communication with a sewer must comply with s.109 of the Act. The undertaker may, as a condition of the permission, require that the sewer or drain to connect with the public sewer (or lateral) be vested in it by virtue of a declaration under s.102.

The Flood and Water Management Act 2010 introduced additional provisions into the 1991 Act by inserting a new Section 106A (s.32 & Schedule 3 of the 2010 Act). This applies to a drainage system whose construction required approval under Schedule 3 to the Flood and Water Management Act 2010 (sustainable urban drainage).

A person may exercise the right under section 106(1) in respect of surface water only if —

a   The construction of the drainage system was approved under that Schedule
b   The proposals for approval included a proposal for communication with
    the public sewer

Where this condition is satisfied, the connection may not be refused under
Section 106(4) or on the grounds that the drainage system absorbs water from
more than one set of premises or sewer, or from land that is neither a premises
nor a sewer.

It is an offence to connect to a public sewer or lateral without prior notice
(or before the expiry of the 21-day notice), and the person responsible will be
liable to a fine not exceeding level 4 on the standard scale.

Within 14 days of receipt of the notice from the owner or occupier, the
undertaker (WaSC) may give notice that they will make the communication
themselves; otherwise, the owner or occupier can make the connection. Where
the undertaker makes the connection, they can charge a payment.

The Building Act 1984[13] (discussed in more detail below) however says
that where plans of a building or of an extension of a building are, in accordance with building regulations, the local authority, or on appeal, a magistrates'
court, may require a proposed drain to connect with a sewer where that sewer is
within 100 ft[14] of the site of the building or, in the case of an extension, the site
either of the extension or of the original building and is at a level that makes it
reasonably practicable to construct a drain to communicate with it. A drain may
be required to be made to connect with a sewer that is not within the distance
above if the authority undertakes to bear so much of the expenses reasonably
incurred in constructing, maintaining and repairing it. If there is a dispute as to
the amount of a payment to be made to a person, that question may, on application, be determined by a magistrates' court, or it may be referred to arbitration.

Any question arising between a local authority and the person who has de-
posited the plans as to whether a proposed drain is to be connected with a sewer
may, on the application of that person, be determined by a magistrates' court.

This section does not apply to works in connection with which approval is
required in accordance with Schedule 3 to the Flood and Water Management
Act 2010 (sustainable drainage).

The power to communicate with the public sewer is a right, not a duty,
and neither the local authority nor the undertaker can require the owner or
occupier of existing premises to communicate with the public sewer unless
it can be shown that satisfactory provision has not been made for drainage
of the building and that the only satisfactory means of doing so would be
to communicate with the public sewer. This would be a matter for the local
authority to decide.

Where, for example, premises are drained into a cesspit that is in good
order and adequate for the purpose, neither the LA nor undertaker can require
the cesspit to be abolished and a connection made to the sewer unless they

offer to pay the costs involved (see s.113 of the WIA'91). Nor would the LA be able to refuse to cleanse or empty the cesspool as a means of putting pressure on the owner of the premises to get them to communicate with a sewer (under s.45(5) of EPA'90).

In *Barratt Homes Ltd v Dwr Cymru (Welsh Water)* [2009] UKSC 13 on appeal from [2008] EWCA 1552 in the Supreme Court, the principal issue raised was whether it was the property owner or the sewerage undertaker who was entitled to determine the point at which the property owner's drain or sewer is to connect to the public sewer. The developer had applied for planning consent for a new housing estate, indicating that connection to the sewer would be at one point. The sewerage undertaker was concerned about overloading of the system and wanted connection further down the public sewer, and planning permission was granted subject to a condition requiring the submission and approval of a scheme of foul and surface water drainage to be completed before the buildings were occupied. The appellant served a notice on the sewerage undertaker under s.106, indicating it would make the connection at the original point on the sewer. The sewerage undertaker had then encased the original proposed connection point in concrete and wanted a connection 400 mm downstream. By a majority verdict of four to one, the Supreme Court dismissed the appeal of Dwr Cymru (Welsh Water) and upheld the Court of Appeal decision, which found that the right of an individual to connect their drain to a public sewer should not be fettered. The Court of Appeal and Supreme Court acknowledged the practical difficulties placed upon water authorities by Section 106 of the Act; their decision was guided by the fact that planning authorities are in a position to support the public water authorities.

The Supreme Court noted that, since the building of a development requires planning permission under the Town and Country Planning Act 1990, planning authorities are able to make planning permission conditional upon the WaSC first taking steps to ensure that the public sewer can accommodate any increased flow. This seems to be saying that the local planning authority has power that the WaSC lacks.

Power to alter drainage

Under s.113, a WaSC may close any existing drain or sewer connecting with a public sewer or cesspool, fill in any such cesspool, and do any work necessary for these purposes. Such work is at the undertaker's expense, and the power is only exercisable in the following circumstances:

*   The drain or sewer in question, although sufficient for the premises, is either not adapted to the sewerage system in the area or, in the opinion of the authority, is otherwise objectionable

- Before exercising such power, the undertaker must first provide, in a position convenient to the owner of the premises, a drain or sewer that effectually drains the premises and communicates with a public sewer
- Notice of the undertaker's proposal must be given to the owner of the premises in question, and if aggrieved so far as the position or sufficiency of the proposed drain or sewer to be provided, may refer the matter to the Director (Ofwat)

Discharges into sewers

Under s.111, it is an offence to throw, empty, or suffer to permit to be thrown or emptied, or to pass into any public sewer, or into any drain or sewer connecting with a public sewer, any of:

- Any matter likely to injure the sewer or drain, interfere with the free flow of its contents, or adversely affect the treatment of its contents
- Any chemical refuse or waste steam or any liquid of a temperature higher than 110°F (67°C), being refuse or steam or a liquid that, when so heated, is either alone or in combination with the contents of the sewer or drain, dangerous, the cause of a nuisance, or prejudicial to health
- Any petroleum spirit (including oil from petroleum, coal, shale peat, or other bituminous substances) or carbide of calcium

Provisions on trade effluent discharges to sewers that were originally in the Public Health (Drainage of Trade Premises) Act 1937 can now be found in the WIA'91 in s.118. The occupier of any trade premises in the area of a sewerage undertaker may only discharge any trade effluent proceeding from those premises into the undertaker's public sewers with the WaSC's consent. Nothing authorises the discharge of any effluent into a public sewer other than by means of a drain or sewer. It is an offence to discharge trade effluent without consent.

Discharges of trade effluent containing certain substances or from certain processes to sewers are also addressed via the environmental permitting regime. In the case of processes requiring a permit under the environmental permitting regime, they may be subject to dual control by the WaSCs and the environmental regulatory agencies, i.e., Environment Agency (England and Wales), Scottish Environmental Protection Agency, and the Northern Ireland Environment Agency. In addition, dual control is also applied in England and Wales for discharges of "Special Category Effluent", as prescribed under the Trade Effluent (Processes and Substances) Regulations.[15]

Trade effluent consents may include conditions on the sewer or sewers into which the trade effluent may be discharged and also the nature or composition of the trade effluent that may be discharged; the maximum quantity of trade effluent that may be discharged on any one day; the highest rate at which trade effluent may be discharged, and the period or periods of the day during which the trade effluent may be discharged from the trade premises into the sewer. Other conditions may exclude all condensing water from the discharge; limitations on any specified constituent of the trade effluent; and the temperature of the trade effluent at discharge. There will also be charges for the reception of the trade effluent into the sewer and for the disposal of the effluent. The conditions may also relate to the provision of access for sampling the effluent, measuring flow rates, and keeping records. The WaSCs levy a charge for trade effluent consents, and this was considered in the Court of Appeal in *Boots UK Limited v Severn Trent Water Limited* [2018] EWCA Civ 2795, where Boots unsuccessfully appealed against a decision that the WaSc was entitled to levy metered charges on the whole of the mixed liquid of its discharge, not just that part that was trade effluent.

The conditions usually, as a minimum, include prohibitions on the discharge of certain materials such as oils, fats, and flammable solvents and also set limits for parameters such as suspended solids, pH, Chemical Oxygen Demand, and flowrate.

Water and Flood Management Act 2010

Reference has already been made to this legislation and the introduction of legislative provisions on sustainable drainage. Schedule 3 of the 2010 Act also introduced standards for the design, construction, maintenance, and operation of new rainwater drainage systems and an 'approving body'. While the Act proposed to establish a SuDS approving body (SAB) at the county and unitary level, the Schedule establishing a SAB has not yet been brought into force in England, and the National Planning Policy Framework was amended to require (where appropriate) the delivery of SuDS for major developments. It was the intention that the SAB would have responsibility for the approval of proposed drainage systems in new developments and redevelopments (in accordance with the National Standards for Sustainable Drainage). The body, which would generally have been a unitary, county, or county borough local authority, would be required to approve most types of rainwater drainage systems before any construction work with drainage implications could start. Where the system affects the drainage of more than one property, the approving body would be required to adopt and maintain the system upon satisfactory completion. There are amendments to s.106 of WIA'91 to make the right to connect surface water to the public sewer conditional on the SAB approving the drainage of the site. Schedule 3 also requires the SAB to adopt and maintain approved SuDS that serve more than one property.

In Wales, from 7 January 2019, the Welsh Government has introduced Schedule 3 of the Flood and Water Management Act 2010. From this date, all new developments of more than one building and/or where the construction area is 100 m² or more will require SuDS for surface water. The SuDS must be designed and built in accordance with Statutory SuDS Standards published by Welsh Ministers, and SuDS schemes must be approved by the SAB before construction work begins. The requirement for SAB approval and adoption agreements for surface water drainage applies only to new developments and is not retrospective. Defra has carried out a review of Schedule 3,[16] and this review recommends that the government act and implement Schedule 3 to the Flood and Water Management Act 2010. However, SuDS should not be delivered purely via the planning system or newly created SAB but with the unitary authority or, if there is not one for the area, then the county council as approving bodies. The argument will be that this will ensure a consistent and more effective approach to using SuDS, but given the restrictions on local government resources, it is questionable whether this will "help address the impacts of climate change, urbanisation, and increasing population while achieving multiple benefits such as reducing surface water flood risk, improving water quality, and harvesting rainwater".

The successful implementation of Schedule 3 will require professionals with the skills and knowledge to design, construct, assess, and maintain SuDS – are these there in all relevant authorities. The review does recommend action to ensure there is sufficient access to the right skills and capabilities to deliver and maintain SuDS, but it remains to be seen if this happens.

The Act places a duty on the relevant Minister to publish national standards about how drainage systems should be designed, constructed, maintained, and operated for the purpose of implementing sustainable drainage. These were published in 2015 for England and 2018 for Wales.[17]

When approving an application for new drainage (construction of a new sewer), the Approving Body may require the applicant to deposit a non-performance bond as a condition of granting approval. The value of the bond will be decided by the Approving Body, but it cannot exceed the best estimate of how much it will cost to build the drainage system in line with the approved proposals. If the Approving Body certifies that the drainage system has not been constructed in accordance with approved proposals or is unlikely to be completed, it may issue a certificate leading to forfeit of the bond.

Section 21 of the Act requires lead local flood authorities (the unitary authority or county council) to establish and maintain a register of structures or features that may significantly affect a flood risk in their area and also a record of information about such structures and features, including ownership and state of repair.

Water Act 2014

The WIA 91 required water and sewerage undertakers to agree charging schemes with Ofwat prior to charging their customers. This was seen as an

overly burdensome and regulatory approach, requiring a significant concentration of resources each year. Therefore, this Act repealed this duty and
replaced it with a power for Ofwat to produce charging rules with which
the companies must comply in setting their charge schemes and a power for
Ministers to issue charging guidance to Ofwat that will shape their charging
rules. Alongside this, the Act also allows for the creation of a new charging
scheme for developers and other customers connecting to water and sewerage infrastructure.

The Act also amends the WIA '91 to confirm undertakers have the power
to construct, maintain, and operate drainage systems.

Part 3 of the Act focuses on the environmental permitting regime (see below) and the power to consolidate into that regime the requirements relating to
water abstraction and impoundment licences, flood defence consents, and fish
passage approvals. It contains powers that enable a single set of regulations
covering the existing pollution prevention and control permit requirements
and new regulations for abstraction licences, flood defence consents, and fish
pass approvals. This single set of regulations will enable operators to apply for
one permit rather than multiple permits.

It does also repeal the provisions in the Public Health Act 1936 on local
authority powers to culvert watercourses and ditches.

Pollution Prevention and Control Act 1999

Environmental permitting & CSOs

Sewage (or wastewater) treatment plants are installations that require an
environmental permit under this Act and the associated regulations.[18] They
are A1 installations and so subject to controls enforced by the Environment
Agency as "water discharge activities". The permits are subject to conditions, and in this case, require the WaSCs to construct and maintain sewerage systems according to their best technical knowledge not entailing
excessive cost. This includes limiting pollution from storm overflows. To
achieve this, operators have to identify those that need improvement. The
permits outline when they can be used as well as how they should be monitored and managed.

Enforcement by the EA and the powers available are considered in the
next chapter.

It should be noted that the environmental permitting regime replaced the
provisions of s.85 of the Water Resources Act 1991 and offences relating to
the pollution of controlled waters. In a case under the 1991 Act, a private
prosecution was brought even though the courts thought the EA should have
brought the case.[19]

Discharges to sewer

As has already been mentioned, where there are discharges to sewers from prescribed processes (other than domestic sewage), there is dual control with the Environment Agencies, and the sewerage undertaker will therefore be involved.

Environment Act 2021

Section 1 provides for regulations to set long-term targets in respect of any matter that relates to the natural environment or people's enjoyment of the natural environment. Water is one of the priority areas.

Section 8 says the Secretary of State must prepare an environmental improvement plan for significantly improving the natural environment in the period to which the plan relates. That period must not be shorter than 15 years. With an annual report on the implementation of the current improvement plan.

Chapter 2 established the Office for Environmental Protection (see Chapter 1), and Part 5 of the Act deals with water. Section 80 introduces a new s.104A into WIA'91 under which the Secretary of State must prepare a plan for the purposes of reducing discharges from the storm overflows of sewerage undertakers whose area is wholly or mainly in England and reducing the adverse impacts (both to the environment and public health) of those discharges. "Reducing discharges" of sewage includes reducing both the frequency and duration of discharges and reducing the volume of the discharges.

A new s.141DA of the 1991 Act, where there is a discharge from a storm overflow of a sewerage undertaker whose area is wholly or mainly in England, the undertaker must publish the following information:

- That there has been a discharge from the storm overflow
- The location of the storm overflow
- When the discharge began
- When the discharge ended

Under a new s.141DB of the 1991 Act, the WaSCs have to monitor continuously the water upstream and downstream of a Combined Sewer Outfall (CSO). The new Section 141DC requires a WaSC in England to secure a progressive reduction in the adverse impacts of discharges from the undertaker's storm overflows. Section 84 of the Act requires the Secretary of State to prepare a report by September 2022 on the actions that would be needed to eliminate discharges from the storm overflows of sewerage undertakers whose areas are wholly or mainly in England.

Environmental Protection Act 1990

Part III and statutory nuisance

Section 79 of the 1990 Act says that premises in such a state as to be prejudicial to health or a nuisance are statutory nuisances. Thus, it can be argued that drainage, sewerage, or drainage problems that lead to raw sewage entering the property or WC pans overflowing would fall within the scope of a statutory nuisance. However, as the *East Riding of Yorkshire* case shows, sewers themselves are not premises. Relevant cases are considered in more detail later, but as a result of the decisions in these cases, it is likely that Part III of the Act will be of limited value, although it can be useful in specific instances in and around dwellings as public sewers themselves have been held not to be "premises". In the *Bradford* case discussed later, it was accepted that premises affected by sewage were in such a state as to be a statutory nuisance; the issue was whether the source of the sewage was a public sewer, and therefore the WaSC was responsible for the state of the premises affected.

Section 79 also includes the provision that any accumulation or deposit that is prejudicial to health or a nuisance and any insects emanating from relevant industrial, trade, or business premises and being prejudicial to health or a nuisance will be statutory nuisances. At first sight, these provisions may not seem relevant, but as will be seen in discussing relevant cases, they might be of use to local authorities in certain circumstances, for example, where sewage and sludge accumulate on land.

The *Hounslow* case,[20] discussed in more detail later in this chapter, does at least mean that, whilst public sewers may not be premises for s.79(1)(a), now at least sewage treatment works are seen as industrial, trade, or business premises for the purposes of s.79(1)(d).

Also, in *R v Carrick DC ex p Shelley,* discussed later, it was clear that sewage debris accumulating on a beach fell within the scope of an accumulation under s.79(1)(e). There had been complaints over a number of years about sewage-related debris finding its way onto the beach.

It is the duty of every local authority to inspect its area from time to time to detect any statutory nuisances that ought to be dealt with under Section 80 below and, where a complaint of a statutory nuisance is made to it by a person living within its area, to take such steps as are reasonably practicable to investigate the complaint.

Where a local authority is satisfied that a statutory nuisance exists or is likely to occur or recur in the area of the authority, they have to serve an abatement notice imposing all or any of the following requirements: Either requiring the abatement of the nuisance or prohibiting or restricting its occurrence or recurrence; and/or requiring the execution of such works and the taking of such other steps as may be necessary for any of those purposes.

Part II waste management

Under Part II, it has been held that sewage is a controlled waste and therefore subject to the Duty of Care; see *R (on the application of Thames Water Utilities Ltd) v Bromley Magistrates' Court* [2008] EWHC 1763 (QB).

Public Health Act 1936

Power of local authority to examine and test drains, etc., believed to be defective

Under Section 48, where it appears to a local authority that there are reasonable grounds for believing that a

> sanitary convenience, drain, private sewer or cesspool is in such a condition as to be prejudicial to health or a nuisance, or that a drain or private sewer communicating... indirectly with a public sewer is so defective as to admit subsoil water, they may examine its condition, and for that purpose may apply any test, other than a test by water under pressure, and, if they deem it necessary, open the ground.

This would include drains that allow rats to escape, and such tests include smoke tests or closed-circuit television to locate the damaged lengths of underground pipe from which rats are escaping.

If on examination the convenience, drain, sewer, or cesspool is found to be in proper condition, the authority shall, as soon as possible, reinstate any ground that has been opened by them and make good any damage done by them.

This provision is as amended by the Water Consolidation (Consequential Provisions) Act 1991. The power of entry is provided by s.287 of the 1936 Act. Once on the land, it is important to act within the powers of the section or within the terms of any agreement with the landowner or other interested person.

Overflowing and leaking cesspools, ditches, etc.

(As amended by Water Act 1989)

Under s.50, if the contents of any cesspool soak away from it or overflow, the local authority may, by notice, require the person by whose act, default, or sufferance the soakage or overflow occurred or continued to execute such works, or to take such steps by periodically emptying the cesspool or otherwise, as may be necessary for preventing the soakage or overflow: Provided that this subsection shall not apply in relation to the effluent from a properly constructed tank for the reception and treatment of sewage if that effluent is of such a character and is so conveyed away and disposed of as not to be prejudicial to health or a nuisance.

Where a notice under this section requires a person to execute works, the provisions of Part XII of this Act with respect to appeals against and the enforcement of notices requiring the execution of works shall apply.

Where a notice requires a person to take any steps other than the execution of works, he shall, if he fails to comply with the notice, be liable to a fine not exceeding level 1 on the standard scale, with a daily penalty not exceeding £2 for each day on which the offence continues after conviction.

Provided that in any proceedings under this subsection, it shall be open to the defendant to question the reasonableness of the authority's requirements.

Section 259 says that any pond, pool, ditch, gutter, or watercourse that is so foul or in such a state as to be prejudicial to health or a nuisance is a statutory nuisance for the purposes of Part 3 of the Environmental Protection Act 1990. As is any part of a water course (non-navigable), which is so choked or silted as to obstruct or impeded, the proper flow of water and thereby cause a nuisance or give rise to conditions that are prejudicial to health. On this, see the *Falmouth and Truro Port Health Authority* case later.

Responsibility and liability fall only on the person through whose act or default the nuisance arises or continues. The local authority has to discover the offender or establish that they have a legal duty to clear the watercourse and have failed to perform that duty. A riparian owner may be under a limited common law duty to clear out a natural stream (may be difficult to prove sufficient act or default), although it will be different if the defendant has created an artificial watercourse or has made artificial that which was natural. What is reasonable for the occupier? (See also s.90 of the Water Resources Act 1990.)

s. 287 Power to enter premises

Subject to the provisions of this section, any authorised officer of a council shall, on producing, if so required, some duly authenticated document showing his authority, have a right to enter any premises at all reasonable hours for the purpose of ascertaining whether there is, or has been, on or in connection with the premises any contravention of the provisions of this Act or of any byelaws or building regulations made under these provisions, being provisions which it is the duty of the council to enforce.

The power also applies for:

• The purpose of ascertaining whether or not circumstances exist that would authorise or require the council to take any action or execute any work under this Act or any such byelaws or building regulations

- For the purpose of taking any action or executing any work authorised or required by this Act or any such byelaws or building regulations, or any order made under this Act, to be taken or executed by the council
- Generally, for the purpose of the performance by the council of their functions under this Act or any such byelaws or building regulations

Provided that admission to any premises not being a factory, or workplace, shall not be demanded as of right unless 24 hours' notice of the intended entry has been given to the occupier.

It is also possible to enter by warrant issued by a Justice of the Peace on sworn information where admission to any premises has been refused, or that refusal is apprehended, or that the premises are unoccupied or the occupier is temporarily absent, or that the case is one of urgency, or that an application for admission would defeat the object of the entry, and there is reasonable ground for entry into the premises for any such purpose as aforesaid.

Public Health Act 1961

Powers to repair drains, etc., and to remedy stopped-up drains, etc.

Under s.17, if it appears to a local authority that a drain, private sewer, water closet, waste pipe, or soil pipe is not sufficiently maintained and kept in good repair and can be sufficiently repaired at a cost not exceeding £250, the local authority may, after giving not less than seven days' notice to the person or persons concerned, cause the drain, private sewer, water closet, or pipe to be repaired. Subject to subsections (7) and (8), the expenses reasonably incurred in so doing can be recovered, so far as they do not exceed £250. They may be recovered from the person or persons concerned in such proportions, if there is more than one such person, as the local authority may determine.

"Person concerned" above means, in relation to a water closet, waste pipe, or soil pipe, the owner or occupier of the premises on which it is situated, and in relation to a drain or private sewer, any person owning any premises drained by means of it, and also, in the case of a sewer, the owner of the sewer.

Under subsection 3, if it appears to a local authority that on any premises a drain, private sewer, water closet, waste pipe, or soil pipe is stopped up, they may, by notice in writing, require the owner or occupier of the premises where the blockage occurs to remedy the defect within 48 hours from the service of the notice. Service of notice is valid; it is sufficient that it appears to the local authority that a drain is blocked on those premises, even if it later transpires that the blockage is on other premises.

If a notice under subsection 3 of this section is not complied with, the local authority may themselves carry out the work necessary to remedy the defect and, subject to subsections 7 and 8, may recover the expenses reasonably incurred in so doing from the person on whom the notice was served (subsection 4).

Where the expenses recoverable by a local authority under subsection (1) or (4) of this section do not exceed £10, the local authority may, if they think fit, remit the payment of the expenses (subsection 5).

In proceedings to recover expenses under this section where the expenses were incurred under subsection 1 of this section, the court shall inquire whether the local authority was justified in concluding that the drain, private sewer, water closet, waste pipe, or soil pipe was not sufficiently maintained and kept in good repair and may inquire whether any apportionment of expenses by the local authority under that subsection was fair. For expenses incurred under subsection 4, the court may inquire whether any requirement contained in a notice served under subsection 3 of this section was reasonable and whether the expenses ought to be borne wholly or in part by some person other than the defendant in the proceedings.

Subsections 7 and 8 provide that the court may make such order concerning the expenses or their apportionment as appears to the court to be just, and where the court determines that the local authority was not justified in concluding that a drain, private sewer, water closet, waste pipe, or soil pipe was not sufficiently maintained and kept in good repair, the local authority shall not recover expenses incurred by them under subsection 1 of this section. The court shall not revise an apportionment unless it is satisfied that all persons affected by the apportionment or by an order made by virtue of subsection 6(b)(ii) have had notice of the proceedings and an opportunity to be heard. It is also important for local authorities to be clear how and why costs have been apportioned.

The provisions of subsection 1 of this section shall not authorise a local authority to carry out works on land belonging to any statutory undertakers and held or used by them for the purposes of their undertaking. However, this limitation does not apply to houses or buildings used as offices or showrooms, other than buildings so used that form part of a railway station.

The provisions of this section shall be without prejudice to Section 59 of the 1984 Act, which empowers a local authority to serve notices as regards defective drains.

A notice under s.17 may be served only on the owner or occupier of the premises at which the blockage occurs, even if the effects are felt elsewhere.

Under s.35 of the Local Government (Miscellaneous Provisions) Act 1976, which also addressed blocked private sewers, the local authority may, by notice, require the owners or occupiers of all premises served by a private sewer (now only those taking surface water to a watercourse) to remove the blockage (time period for compliance is not less than 48 hours). The notice could be served on each of the people who are owners or occupiers of premises served by the sewer, or on such of those people as the authority thinks fit. Where an authority has reasonably incurred expenses in removing an obstruction, it may serve on each of the persons on whom it served notice a further notice:

- Requiring him/her to pay to the authority a sum equal to so much of the expenses as is specified in the further notice
- Specifying the other persons on whom notices in pursuance of this subsection have been or are to be served in respect of the expenses and the amount specified or to be specified in each of those notices

In determining what amounts to specify in notices to be served by the authority in pursuance of this subsection in respect of any expenses, it must have regard to any matters that appear to indicate the cause of the obstruction and, so far as the authority is aware of the obligations, to any obligations to remove the obstruction that arose under agreements between persons on whom the notices are to be served. An appeal against the second notice to recover costs is to the County Court and must be made within six weeks from the date of service of the notice. The ground of appeal is that it would be reasonable for the whole or part of the sum specified in the notice to be paid by some other person who is an owner or occupier of premises served by the sewer in question.

With the transfer of private sewers to the WaSCs, this provision is now of very limited applicability.

Power to cleanse or repair drains

Under s.22, a local authority may, on the application of the owner or occupier of any premises, undertake the cleansing or repair of any drains, water closets, sinks, or gullies in or connected with the premises and may recover from the applicant such reasonable charge, if any, for so doing as they think fit.

Other issues – access to carry out repairs

It has sometimes been problematic when the owner of a drain or private sewer has needed to gain access to the pipeline to carry out a repair and it is running through the land of another person. Again, this should have limited applicability, as once a drain leaves the curtilage, it becomes a public lateral and the responsibility of the WaSC.

The right to lay a drain and cause drainage to flow through it will normally carry with it the ancillary right to enter on the land and effect necessary works of repair, maintenance, or renewal (*Pomfret v Ricroft* (1669) 1 Wms Saunds. 321). It would not allow an increase in the size of the drain. In *Simmons v Midford* [1969] 2 Ch. 415, it was held that a grant of an easement of drainage amounted to an exclusive right to use the line of pipes in question. If the easement is a legal interest, it is enforceable, but it would be necessary to check deeds.

The Access to Neighbouring Land Act 1992 gives a limited right of access to a neighbour's garden/land to carry out "basic preservation works". These works include "the clearance, repair, or renewal of any drain, pipe, or cable so comprised or situate". The right of access given by the Act requires that written notice must be given to neighbouring landowners. However, this right is enforceable by County Court Order (or High Court) and obviates the need for an argument as to entitlement under the deed of ownership.

Building Act 1984

Unsatisfactory drains, etc.

Section 59 of the Building Act 1984 (as amended)[21] provides local authorities with the power to require an owner of a building (as defined in s.126 of the 1984 Act) to remedy a drain, private sewer, or similar apparatus that is insufficient (satisfactory provision has not been made for drainage[22]), prejudicial to health, or a nuisance.

So that if it appears to a local authority that in the case of a building

1   Satisfactory provision has not been, and ought to be, made for drainage (for these purposes, 'drainage' includes the conveyance, by means of a sink and any other necessary appliance, of refuse water and the conveyance of rainwater from roofs)
2   A cesspool, private sewer, drain, soil pipe, rain water pipe, spout, sink, or other necessary appliance provided for the building is insufficient or, in the case of a private sewer or drain communicating directly or indirectly with a public sewer, is so defective as to admit subsoil water
3   A cesspool or other such work or appliance mentioned previously provided for the building is in such a condition as to be prejudicial to health or a nuisance[23]
4   A cesspool, private sewer, or drain formerly used for the drainage of the building but no longer used for it is prejudicial to health or a nuisance

The local authority must by notice require the owner of the building to make satisfactory provision for the drainage of the building, or, as the case may be, require either the owner or the occupier of the building to do such work as may be necessary for renewing, repairing, or cleansing the existing cesspool, sewer, drain, pipe, spout, sink, or other appliance, or for filling up, removing, or otherwise rendering innocuous the disused cesspool, sewer, or drain.

Under subsections 4 and 5, this duty, so far as it empowers a local authority to take action in the cases mentioned in (1) and (2) above, does not apply in relation to a building belonging to statutory undertakers, the Civil Aviation Authority, or a person who holds a licence under the provisions relating to air traffic services and held or used by such a body or person for the purposes of that body's or that person's undertaking, unless it is: (a) a house; or (b) a building used as offices or showrooms and not forming part of a railway station. or in the case of the Civil Aviation Authority, not being on an aerodrome owned by the Authority. The undertaking of a person who holds a licence under Chapter I of Part 1 of the Transport Act 2000 shall be taken to be the person's undertaking as a licence holder. It would seem that s.59 is not available for dealing with a former private sewer that has been transferred to the WaSC after 1 October 2011.

Work can be undertaken by the local authority by agreement with the person(s) served. Any notice shall indicate the nature of the works to be executed and state the time within which they are to be executed.

Here, "cesspool" includes a settlement tank or other tank for the reception or disposal of foul matter from buildings (s.90 Public Health Act 1936);

'Owner' means the person for the time being receiving the rack rent of the premises in connection with which the word is used, whether on his own account or as agent or trustee for another person, or who would so receive it if those premises were let at a rack rent (Building Act 1984 s.126). 'Rack rent', in relation to property, means a rent that is not less than two-thirds of the rent at which the property might reasonably be expected to let from year to year, free from all usual tenant's rates and taxes, and deducting from it the probable average annual cost of the repairs, insurance, and other expenses, if any, necessary to maintain the property in a state to command such rent: s 126. 'Premises' includes buildings, land, easements, and hereditaments of any tenure.

Section 99 requires that the notice shall indicate the nature of the works to be executed and state the time within which they are to be executed.

Subject to any right of appeal to the magistrate's court (as provided by s.102), if the person required by such a notice to execute works fails to execute them within the time limited by the notice, the local authority may themselves execute the works and recover from that person the expenses reasonably incurred by them in doing so. Without prejudice to that power, that person is also liable on summary conviction to a fine not exceeding level 4 on the standard scale and to a further fine not exceeding £2 for each day on which the default continues after conviction.

Grounds of appeal under s.102 are

- That the notice or requirement is not justified by the terms of the provision under which it purports to have been given
- That there has been some informality, defect, or error in, or in connection with, the notice
- That the authority has refused unreasonably to approve the execution of alternative works, or that the works required by the notice to be executed are otherwise unreasonable in character or extent, or are unnecessary

- That the time within which the works are to be executed is not reasonably sufficient for the purpose
- That the notice might lawfully have been served on the occupier of the premises in question instead of on the owner, or on the owner instead of on the occupier, and that it would have been equitable for it to have been so served
- Where the works are for the common benefit of the premises in question and other premises, some other person, being the owner or occupier of the premises to be benefited, ought to contribute towards the expenses of executing any works required

If an appeal is based on the ground of some informality, defect, or error in or in connection with the notice, then the court shall dismiss the appeal if it is satisfied that the informality, defect, or error was not a material one.

As to the recovery of expenses, where a local authority has incurred expenses and the owner of the premises is liable for repaying those expenses, whether the work has been done by agreement or in default of compliance with a notice, they, together with interest from the date of service of a demand for the expenses, may be recovered by the authority.

- From the person who is the owner of the premises at the date on which the works are completed or
- If he has ceased to be the owner of the premises before the date on which a demand for the expenses is served, either from him or from the person who is the owner at the date on which the demand is served.

and, from the date of the completion of the works, the expenses and interest accrued thereon are a charge on the premises until recovered.

A local authority, for the purposes of enforcing a charge, has all the same powers and remedies under the Law of Property Act 1925 as if they were mortgagees by deed having powers of sale and lease, of accepting surrenders of leases, and of appointing a receiver. The rate of interest chargeable under subsection (1) above is such a reasonable rate as the authority may determine. A sum that a local authority is entitled to recover under this Act and with respect to which recovery provision is not made by any other section of this Act may be recovered as a simple contract debt in any court of competent jurisdiction.

Where a person has been given a notice in relation to which Section 102 applies (appeal against a notice requiring works such as s.59), and the local authority takes proceedings against him for the recovery of expenses, it is not open to him to raise any question that could have been raised on an appeal.

It was the case that where part of the sewer or drain was defective and part was not, the authority may serve notice only on those owners or occupiers of buildings served by the sewer up to the point where it is defective (*Swansea City Council v Jenkins* [1994] C.O.D. 398). Now any sewer will be the responsibility of the WaSC unless it takes only surface water and discharges it to a watercourse. It should be noted that the term "prejudicial to health or a nuisance" has the same meaning as in the statutory nuisance provisions in Part III of the EPA'90, previously considered.

It has been demonstrated that the law determining ownership of sewers is complex, even if, in theory at least, things have been simplified with the transfer of private sewers. If works are carried out on a public sewer by a person acting under the misapprehension that they were repairing his own sewer as required by such a notice, they may recover the expenses incurred from the Council or undertaker (*Andrew v St Olaves Board* [1898] 1 Q.B. 775).

Section 60 requires that a pipe for conveying rainwater from a roof shall not be used for the purpose of conveying the soil or drainage from a sanitary convenience; the soil pipe from a water closet shall be properly ventilated; and a pipe for conveying surface water from premises shall not be permitted to act as a ventilating shaft to a drain or sewer conveying foul water. If it appears to the local authority that there is on any premises a contravention of any provision of this section, they may, by notice, require the owner or occupier of those premises to execute such work as may be necessary to remedy the matter.

It should be noted that only the owner of premises can be served under s.59 to make proper provision, but under s.60, either the owner or the occupier may be required to take action. These provisions only apply to buildings, not all types of premises. Under Section 98, if, on a complaint made by the owner of premises, it appears to a magistrates' court that the occupier of those premises prevents the owner from executing any work that he is required to execute under s.59, the court may order the occupier to permit the execution of the work.

Notice of repairs, etc.

This is a provision that seems to be commonly ignored. By virtue of s.61, no person shall, other than in an emergency, repair, reconstruct, or alter the course of an underground drain that communicates with a sewer or with a cesspool or other receptacle for drainage. In an emergency where works have been executed without notice, the drain (or sewer) should not be covered up without giving the local authority at least 24 hours' of notice the intention to do so.

While any such work is being executed, all persons concerned shall permit the proper officer, or any other authorised officer, of the local authority to have free access to the work.

Failure to comply with this section makes the person responsible liable on summary conviction to a fine not exceeding level 3 on the standard scale.

This section does not apply to drains or sewers constructed by, or belonging to, a railway company running under, across, or along their railway, or drains or sewers constructed by, or belonging to, dock undertakers, as is situated in or on land of the undertakers that is held or used by them for the purposes of their undertaking.

Disconnecting drains

Section 62 provides that where a drain is no longer to be used, the local authority may require it to be disconnected and sealed at such points as it may reasonably specify. The Magistrates Court will determine what is reasonable. However, no such work can be required of a person who has no right of access to the land on which the work is required. It is an offence to knowingly fail to comply with a local authority requirement and to fail to give a minimum of 48 hours prior notice of the commencement of work to comply. This cab can also be relevant when it comes to dealing with rat infestations, which may be the result of redundant lengths of drain.

Section 80 of the Building Act applies to any demolition of the whole or part of a building except:

a   A demolition in pursuance of a demolition order [or obstructive building order] made under [Part IX of the Housing Act 1985 as amended]
b   A demolition of an internal part of a building, where the building is occupied and it

is intended that it should continue to be occupied, or of a building that has a cubic content (as ascertained by external measurement) of not more than 1,750 cubic feet, or, where a greenhouse, conservatory, shed, or prefabricated garage forms part of a larger building, of that greenhouse, conservatory, shed, or prefabricated garage and certain agricultural buildings

This section requires that no person shall begin a demolition to which this section applies unless notice of intention has been given to the local authority and either the local authority has given notice to him/her under Section 81 or the relevant period has expired.

A person who contravenes section 80(2) above is liable on summary conviction to a fine not exceeding level 4 on the standard scale.

Under s.81, the local authority may also serve a notice in writing requiring persons engaged in the demolition of buildings to disconnect and seal any sewers or drains in or under the buildings at such points as are reasonable. They may also require the removal of such conduits and any connecting drains or sewers to be sealed. At least 48 hours' notice of compliance with such a requirement is required. Work cannot be required beyond the demolition site if the person engaged in demolition lacks the relevant property rights. The local authority has the power to carry out work in default of compliance and recover the costs. Use of s.81 disapplies s.61.

The improper construction or repair of a water closet or drain

Section 63 requires that if a water closet, drain, or soil pipe is so constructed or repaired as to be prejudicial to health or a nuisance, the person who undertook or executed the construction or repair is liable on summary conviction to a fine not exceeding level 1 on the standard scale, unless he shows that the prejudice to health or nuisance could not have been avoided by the exercise of reasonable care.

Further, under subsection 2, a person charged with an offence under this section (hereafter referred to as "the original defendant") is entitled, upon information duly laid by him and on giving to the prosecutor not less than three clear days' notice of his intention, to have any other person, being his agent or servant, to whose act or default he alleges that the offence was due, brought before the court at the time appointed for the hearing of the charge. If, after the commission of the offence has been proved, the original defendant proves that the offence was due to the act or default of that other person, that other person may be convicted of the offence, and if the original defendant further proves that he used all due diligence to secure that the water closet, drain, or soil pipe in question was so constructed or repaired as not to be prejudicial to health or a nuisance, he shall be acquitted of the offence.

Where the original defendant seeks to avail himself of the defence provided by subsection 2, the prosecutor as well as the person whom the original defendant charges with the offence has the right to cross-examine the original defendant, if he gives evidence, and any witness called by him in support of his pleas, and to call rebutting evidence, and the court may make such order as it thinks fit for the payment of costs by any party to the proceedings to any other party to them.

As will be seen from the consideration of recent cases in the following section, the statutory nuisance provision of Part III of the EPA'90 has not been of much assistance to local authorities in trying to deal with public sewer problems. Yet premises in such a state as to be prejudicial to health or a nuisance as a consequence of sewerage problems leading to, for example, raw sewage entering the property or WC pans overflowing would fall within the scope of a statutory nuisance.

The *Hounslow* case does at least mean that, whilst public sewers may not be premises for s.79(1)(a), now at least sewage treatment works are seen as industrial, trade, or business premises for the purposes of s.79(1)(d).

Under Part II of the Act, it has also been held that sewage is a controlled waste and therefore subject to the Duty of Care; see *R (on the application of Thames Water Utilities Ltd) v Bromley Magistrates' Court* [2008] EWHC 1763 (QB); see later.

Highways Act 1980

Drains that take surface water from a highway and that serve no other purpose will normally be vested in the highway authority by s.263 of the Highways Act 1980. This is usually the County Council or metropolitan districts outside London; the main exceptions are trunk and special roads vested in the Secretary of State (Highways Agency). A drain on the highway is the responsibility of the highway authority only if it is not a public sewer, forms part of the road or highway, or is vested in the highway authority.

Where a highway drain also conveys foul or surface water from premises in the vicinity of the highway, or where it is required to connect drains from premises to the highway drain, it has to be determined whether the highway drain is a public sewer.

Highway drains constructed after 1 October 1937 by the highway authority will be public sewers if they were constructed under some statutory provision relating to the sewering of private streets. They will also be public sewers if constructed before 1 April 1974 by a highway authority that was at the time also the local sanitary authority, and provided that they then drained property(ies) other than that belonging to the local authority.

Such drains, draining the highway alone, or if constructed, whether before or after 1 April 1974, by a highway authority that was not the local sanitary authority, will not be public sewers unless a declaration of vesting has been made by the water authority or the sewerage undertaker.

A highway drain constructed prior to 1 October 1937, which belonged to a highway and the highway authority, which was not the local sanitary authority, was excluded from the definition of sewer in the 1875 Act and so did not vest in the local authority, or now the sewerage undertaker. It seems a drain belonging to the main road vested in the county council as highway authority but transferred to the district council, which was also the sanitary authority, would not become a public sewer.

The fact that surface water flows from a highway drain into a public sewer would not affect the status of the highway drain.

Under s.100(1) of the Act, the highway authority for a highway may, for the purpose of draining it or for the purpose of preventing surface water from flowing onto it, scour, cleanse, and keep open all drains situated in the highway. Note that this is a power, not a duty, and so they cannot be compelled to keep the drain clean. However, they are under an express duty to maintain any highway maintainable at the public expense that is vested in them (ss.41 & 58 Highways Act 1980), and this could be construed as requiring them to maintain any drains that are part of the highway. The defence of non-feasance that was previously available is no longer available to highway authorities because of the duties imposed under ss.41 & 58 and should extend to the maintenance of drains that are part of the highway.

A manhole cover of a public sewer running under the highway is generally treated as part of the sewer, not the highway,[24] unless the drain or sewer itself is a highway drain originally constructed for the purpose of draining the highway alone. Gullies and gratings leading to a public sewer will form part of that sewer (*White v Hindley Local Board* (1875) L.R. 10 Q.B. 219 where the issue was a failure to maintain) unless provided for the sole purpose of draining the highway when they will be part of the highway (*Papworth v Battersea Corporation* (No 2) [1916] 1 KB. 583).

The Flood and Water Management Act 2010 amended Section 115(5) of the WIA'91 (highway drains and sewers) by the addition of "(5A) A sewerage undertaker must accept any use by a highway authority that is in accordance with a drainage system approved under Schedule 3 to the Flood and Water Management Act 2010".

Housing Act 2004

This book is concerned primarily with how sewage can threaten public health, and while much concern arises from sewage discharged into the wider environment, the point has been made that most sewage arises from the home and there can be risks to health closer to accommodation, and the provisions in the 2004 Act reflect that.

Part 1 of the Housing Act 2004 introduces a new method for assessing housing and introduces the concept of category 1 (which local housing authorities will be under a duty to deal with) and category 2 hazards.[25] The category of hazards will be identified by reference to the Housing Health and Safety Rating System (HHSRS), which will be prescribed in secondary legislation. The HHSRS focuses on the risk to health and safety from defects and the hazards arising out of these deficiencies, and using that system, hazards can be defined as Category 1 or Category 2, with the former posing the greater threat. Local housing authorities have a statutory duty to take action on Category 1 hazards. There are two potential hazards relevant to drainage. "Personal hygiene and sanitation" covers the threat of infection and threats to mental health associated with personal hygiene, including personal washing and clothes washing facilities, sanitation, and drainage. Thus, disrepair to the foul or waste-water drainage systems would be considered under this hazard.

The hazard of "Domestic hygiene, pests and refuse" covers deficiencies to the drainage system that could allow pests to enter the premises, which again could include disrepair to the drainage/sewerage system, including inspection chambers.

Some relevant cases

This section reports on a number of cases of interest, some of which are referred to in the earlier parts of the chapter. These reports are intended to illustrate some of the complexities of the legal framework rather than set out any legal analysis; the author is not qualified to provide that.

Marcic v Thames Water Utilities Ltd *All ER (D) 202 (May)* *[2001] and [2002] EWCA Civ 64*

This is an important case that is referred to in several places and is relevant when properties are flooded by sewage.

The plaintiff brought proceedings contending that the flooding constituted a nuisance for which Thames Water was liable as the statutory undertaker responsible for their operation and maintenance and by virtue of duty s.94 of the WIA'91. Liability was also alleged at common law in nuisance and under s.6 of the Human Rights Act (HRA) 1998.

Reference was made to a number of cases, for example, *Glossop v Heston & Isleworth Local Board* [1879] 12 Ch D 102 and *Hesketh v Birmingham Corporation* [1924] 1 K.B. 260. In *Hesketh,* it had been concluded, however, that a local authority is liable for misfeasance but not for non-feasance, and the Court was of the view that the same applies to a statutory undertaker that is not a local authority. Thus, a sewerage undertaker was not liable to a person in its area who suffered damage by flooding where the claim was based on the failure of the undertaker to undertake works to fulfil its statutory duty of drainage of the area.

The duty under s.94 of the WIA'91 is enforceable only by way of an enforcement order made by the Secretary of State or the Director General under s.18. The Act provides that contravention of such an order can give rise to an action by a person who has suffered loss or damage as a result (s.22). In this case, no such order had been made.

Marcic was successful in the High Court in arguing a breach of the HRA 1988, but the Court took the view that the inactivity of the defendant only became unlawful on 2 October 2000, when the HRA 1998 came into force, and the cause of action under s.8(1) of the 1998 Act; the cause of action is a continuing one. Marcic was unsuccessful with the claim based on nuisance.

However, the Court of Appeal heard appeals by both Marcic and Thames Water Utilities from the decision of the High Court. It allowed the appeal by Marcic, who had a "valid claim in nuisance under the common law" and the *Glossop* line of authority referred to above, and the issue of misfeasance and non-misfeasance was no bar to that claim. The Court of Appeal dismissed Thames Water's appeal and held that the company was liable under the HRA 1988 having breached Marcic's rights under Article 8 of the Convention and Article 1 of the first protocol (*Marcic v Thames Water Utilities Ltd* [2002] EWCA Civ 64). This raises the question whether water and sewerage undertakers could be liable in nuisance for rat infestation emanating from public sewers that have not been properly maintained or where there has been no sewer baiting.

Thames Water Utilities subsequently appealed to the House of Lords, and their appeal was successful.[26]

Dwr Cymru Cyfyngedig v Barratt Homes Ltd *[2013]* *EWCA Civ 233*

This was an appeal by the WaSC Dwr Cymru Cyfynngedig ("DCC") against the decision of a Deputy High Court Judge refusing to strike out the claims in nuisance and trespass to goods and also refusing to grant summary judgement to DCC in respect of those claims. There was also a cross-appeal by the respondent, Barratt Homes Limited (BHL), in respect of the judge's ruling that, with the exception of a claim in respect of physical damage to a pipe and its reinstatement, the claim in negligence be struck out.

BHL gave notice pursuant to Section 106, WIA'91 to the defendant DCC of its intention to connect a housing development by its drains to the public sewer at the point. Section 106(4) provides that notice of refusal to permit the communication may be given by the undertaker within 21 days of receiving a notice under Section 106. No such notice of refusal was given by the defendant DCC. B alleged that in June 2008, DCC poured concrete into the claimant's drainage pipe, through which it intended to make the connection to the public sewer pursuant to the Section 106 notice, preventing the connection from taking place or disconnecting the connection. By that date, the claimant had built a total of 38 houses on the development land and was in the course of constructing the school. In addition, the claimant intended to build further houses on the development land pursuant to the planning permission. B claimed to have suffered loss and damage as a result of DCC preventing the connection, in that it had to place a temporary storage tank within the land to receive foul sewage from the houses and the school, which then had to be pumped out and removed by tanker during the period to December 2008.

It was alleged that DCC's conduct amounted to a breach of statutory duty and/or an act of trespass to or wrongful interference with B's drainage pipe and/or a nuisance, which constituted a wrongful interference with B's use and enjoyment of the development land. It is further alleged that DCC "was negligent in that it failed to take reasonable care to prevent injury to the claimant in that it poured concrete into the claimant's pipes and/or prevented the claimant's lawful connection, thereby causing foreseeable loss to the claimant" (B).

In the context of statutes dealing with this issue, the Court was not able to conclude that the policy of the 1991 Act intended to confer a right to compensation for breach of Section 106. This case was distinguished from *Marcic's*. The Appeal was allowed, and the cross-appeal was dismissed.

Oldcorn and another v Southern Water Services Ltd *[2017]* *EWHC 62 (TCC)*[27]

The claimants were the freehold owners of a property that was the subject of surface water flooding on 11 June 2012. The Claimants argued that the flood was caused by the Defendants negligently inserting a Tideflex valve into one of its own pipes, the effect of which was to significantly reduce flow through the pipe, which in turn led to water backing up behind the Tideflex valve and, asserted the Claimants, causing flooding of the Property. The Property was at risk of flooding from both seawater and rainwater owing to its low-lying location and the nature and extent of the drainage installed on the Estate where the property is located.

The following issues fell to be determined (not all discussed here):

i The relevant legal framework to be applied includes the extent, if any, of the Defendants' common law duty to prevent the Property from flooding; whether the Property enjoyed a right of drainage into the Pipe and, if so, the extent of that right; and, if not, the consequences for the Claimants' claim; and whether the Defendants are entitled to take advantage of the so-called common enemy defence

ii The extent of the flooding at the Property

iii Whether the installation of the Tideflex was negligent

iv Whether the Property would have avoided flooding "but for" the presence of the Tideflex

v Quantum

Southern Water submitted that a duty in negligence cannot arise out of the performance of their statutory functions, relying on the cases of *Marcic v Thames Water Utilities Limited, Barratt Homes Ltd v Dwr Cymru Cyfyngedig* [2013] EWCA Civ 233, and *Nicholson v Thames Water* [2014] EWHC 4249.

The allegations made by the Claimants against the Defendants were of misfeasance, namely a positive act of fitting the Tideflex. In those circumstances, it seemed to HHJ McKenna that the duty of care was not subject to the qualification of the measured duty; rather, the Defendants were to be held to the standard of the reasonable water authority.

It was held that the Defendants did owe the Claimants a duty of care in nuisance and negligence; the standard of care was that of the reasonable water authority, and this was not a case where the Defendants could rely on the common enemy rule.

One issue was that the Chamber Tidal Flap was missing in June 2011. What is not clear and was disputed was for how long it was missing. It was submitted on behalf of the Claimants that it was most probably missing at the time of the 2009 flood and might well have been missing since August 2008, when seawater flooding was reported. The Judge accepted the force of the submissions made on the Claimants' behalf and concluded that the weight of the evidence suggested that the flap was indeed missing for a prolonged period of time, which itself supported the Claimants' submissions as to a history of poor maintenance.

On the totality of the evidence, a reasonable statutory sewerage undertaker in the position of the Defendants would have carried out an assessment of the risk of installing a Tideflex. Any such assessment would have established that it posed a substantial restriction to the surface water flows and should not have been installed unless and until a proper evaluation of the respective risks was undertaken and an informed judgement made. HHJ McKenna was of the view that this was not done.

To succeed in the claim, the claimants had to prove that the negligence had resulted in the flooding of their property. They relied on a highly experienced expert who had created a hydraulic model of the incident. The defendant relied upon an expert who, in turn relied upon a model created not by him but by the defendants themselves. The Judge disregarded the defendants' evidence as a result of this and the criticisms levied at it by the claimant's expert. That said, the Judge also felt that the claimants' expert evidence on causation fell short of discharging the burden of proof.

The upshot was that, as a result of the numerous concessions and criticisms of the evidence, the Judge held he could not be satisfied on the balance of probabilities that, but for the installation of the Tideflex valve, the property would not have flooded. The claim was therefore dismissed despite the finding of negligence on behalf of the defendants.

Regina v Carrick District Council Ex Parte Shelley and Another: QBD 15 April 1996 Lexis Citation 2077 95 LGR 620, [1996] JPL 857, The Times 15 April 1996

In this case, there were accumulations and deposits on a public beach and about one kilogram per day of material that included sanitary towels, condoms, and weed. This was considered to be prejudicial to health. The presence of this material was capable of amounting to a statutory nuisance, even though there was no evidence that ill health had been caused.

The case itself is an application for judicial review of a decision of the Carrick District Council made by the Environmental and Community Services Committee on 20 June 1995, whereby they declined to serve an abatement notice under s.80 of the Environmental Protection Act 1990 ("the Act") in respect of the beach on the north Cornish coast. Above the high water mark, the beach was owned by the District Council. Between high and low water, it is owned by the Duchy of Cornwall and leased to the National Trust.

In 1995, following a report from the Environmental Health Officer, the relevant council committee resolved not to take any action under the Act, but to continue monitoring the situation and to write to the Secretary of State with respect to some requirements of the then National Rivers Authority.

S79(1)(e) of the Environmental Protection Act 1990 includes "any accumulation or deposit that is prejudicial to health or a nuisance". The section makes it the duty of every local authority to cause its area to be inspected from time to time to detect any statutory nuisances that ought to be dealt with. The Council had not proceeded because it was considered that the National Rivers Authority was the appropriate body to secure a remedy by requiring better treatment by South West Water.

An order for mandamus was sought so as to order the Council to issue an abatement notice, on the basis that that was the only reasonable view they could take of the evidence. However, the Court held that this went too far. There is no way in which the Court can reach a conclusion on that or say that there is only one reasonable view that the Authority could reach. It seemed to Carnwath J, subject to any submissions, that the appropriate remedy was a declaration that the resolution of 20 June 1995 was not a valid discharge of the Authority's duty under s.80 of the Act. Thus, given such a declaration, the Authority should accept that it is under an obligation to reconsider that resolution.

Carnwath J had "some considerable sympathy for the Authority's position". The evidence showed that Carrick and its officers had taken their responsibilities for the beach seriously, and had been diligent in trying to secure action to improve conditions in the sea and on the beach. They were "hampered by the fact that the practical responsibility for improving matters rested with the Water Authority, the NRA, and the Department of the Environment". The delay caused by the WaSC's appeal against requirements by the NRA "put Carrick in a very difficult position". "Their desire not to get involved in a costly battle in the Magistrates Court when the same issue is being considered by the Secretary of State and should, one have thought, have been decided long ago" was understandable.

The upshot was that once satisfied that a statutory nuisance existed the local authority was obliged to serve an abatement notice even where another regulatory agency was involved.

The application was allowed.

R v Falmouth and Truro Port Health Authority, ex parte South West Water Limited *[2000] EWCA Civ J0330-10*

This case has probable greater importance for environmental health in the matter of the degree of consultation it would be advisable for an enforcing authority to take prior to serving a statutory nuisance abatement notice. The case involved an application for judicial review of decisions made on 11 May and 1 July 1998 by Falmouth and Truro Port Health Authority to serve an abatement notice on South West Water Limited under Section 80 of the Environmental Protection Act 1990.

The abatement notice alleged that sewage discharges into a watercourse, which was part of an estuary, had caused a statutory nuisance contrary to Section 259(1)(a) of the Public Health Act 1936 as amended by the Environmental Protection Act 1990. South West Water Limited argued that Falmouth and Truro Port Health Authority had a duty to consult prior to serving the notice arising either out of the Authority's duty to investigate complaints of nuisance under Section 79(1) of the Environmental Protection Act 1990 or under the common law principle of procedural fairness. The judge held that an enforcing authority is not under a duty to consult an alleged perpetuator prior to serving that person with an abatement notice.

The Authority had, however, in this case, approached South West Water Limited to enquire what steps South West Water Limited would take to resolve the dispute. The judge indicated that this gave rise to a legitimate expectation of consultation, which, if not carried through, could make the issuing of an abatement notice susceptible to judicial review.

South West Water Limited also submitted that the estuary did not constitute a watercourse within the meaning of Section 259(1)(a) of the Public Health Act 1936, and therefore the notice was ultra vires and invalid. The judge agreed with this interpretation, stating that, on the wording, Section 259(1)(a) applied to a limited area of water and could not include an estuary. The judge also held that the abatement notice was invalid as it failed to specify the works necessary to abate the nuisance. On these grounds, the court upheld South West Water Limited's application and held the abatement notice to be invalid.

(Reported in Times Law Reports, 6 May 1999)

Bradford Metropolitan District Council v Yorkshire Water Services Ltd *All ER (D) 49 (Sep) [2001]*

In this case, the complexities of the law and the importance of both the status of a pipeline and ownership with respect to maintenance were considered. Here, Lord Justice Brooke and Mr Justice Newman held that a drainage system that served only one house and a road did not constitute a "sewer" or "public sewer", as it was not a public sewer within the meaning of the Public Health Act 1875 on 1 October 1937. The issue was sewage flooding a property, although the new property that was flooded was not served by the pipe in question, it was accepted that a statutory nuisance existed. The sewerage undertaker had referred the complaint to the Council, and joint investigations showed that the system was blocked in front of the house. The local authority had served an abatement notice under Section 80 of the Environmental Protection Act 1990 on Yorkshire Water, complaining about the deposit of sewage from a public sewer at the property. The sewerage undertaker successfully appealed against the notice. Bradford MDC appealed that decision.

Hearing Bradford MDC's appeal, the Divisional Court referred to a number of cases to help with the interpretation of the definition of Section 4 of the 1875 Act and what constitutes drains and sewers (*Acton Local Board v Baten* (1884) Ch D 283, *Wincanton Rural District Council v Parsons* [1905] 2 KB 34, *Blackdown Properties Ltd v Ministry of Housing and Local Government* [1967] 1 Ch 115 (referred to earlier in Chapter 1), and *British Railways Board v Tonbridge and Malling District Council* [1982] JPL 310). These relate to the "purpose" test for deciding whether a pipe is a drain or sewer. A plan from 1885 showed that there were two properties one of which Turf House still existed but had its own drainage system draining into a public sewer to the rear of the property. There was also a farmhouse, and outside the curtilage of that farmhouse was a drain that ran from a street gulley in the lane to the public sewer at the back. It drained the farmhouse as well as the street gulley, and it had been held by the deputy district judge that because the pipe served only the farmhouse and street gulley on 1 October 1937 it was a drain, not a sewer.

The Divisional Court was of the view that the original purpose of the gulley in the lane was to protect a farmhouse from flooding, not to drain the lane. It was built by a private person for private persons and did not take water from the frontage of Turf House, the original property. Again, it was held that the pipe was therefore not a public sewer just because, on 1 October 1937, it took water from both the farmhouse and the lane. The position would, it seems, have been different if the local authority had adopted it in the past. In any event, a sewer is not "premises" for the purposes of s.79(1)(a) of the 1990 Act, (*R v Parlby* (1889) 22 QBD 520) and *East Riding of Yorkshire Council v Yorkshire Water Services* [2000] COD 446 Env.L.R.7) (considered below).

The judges did suggest that a highway, including an unadopted street, is capable of constituting a "premise" within the meaning of Section 4 of the 1875 Act, but this was of no help to the appellants in this case because of the original purpose of the pipe.

Section 102(1)(a) of the WIA'91 Act gives the sewerage undertaker the power to adopt sewers and disposal works situated within their area or serving part of their area. Under Section 102(2), the owner of a sewer can apply to the sewerage undertaker to request that it adopt the sewer. Whilst the undertaker may agree to do this, it is not legally obliged to do so. In deciding whether or not to adopt a sewer, section 102(5) requires the undertaker to have regard to all the circumstances of the case and must take account of specific factors, which include the method of construction and state of repair, its adaptability to the existing or proposed general sewerage system, whether the sewer is constructed under a highway, the number of buildings that the sewer is intended to serve, and the likelihood of it serving additional buildings (section 102(5)(d)).

East Riding of Yorkshire Council v Yorkshire Water Services Ltd,
Queens Bench Division, 24 March 2000, [2000] Env.L.R 7

What came before the Deputy Stipendiary Magistrate was an appeal against that abatement notice. At a hearing on 22 February 1999, two preliminary issues were identified. Firstly, whether the sewer was a public sewer, and secondly, whether the sewer, if found to be a public sewer, was capable of being premises within the meaning of s.79(1)(a). The issue as to whether the sewer was a public sewer had to be resolved by evidence but was not the subject of the appeal, although the Deputy Stipendiary Magistrate concluded that the sewer was a public sewer.

The issue in the appeal related to the second preliminary issue, namely whether a public sewer is capable of being premises. That is, whether a public sewer could be premises for the purposes of s.79(1)(a) of the Environmental Protection Act 1990? The Deputy Stipendiary Magistrate concluded that the public sewer was not a premises within the meaning of s.79(1)(a).

On behalf of the Appellant, a number of submissions were made. The first was that the subterranean pipes constituting the sewer in this case amounted to a structure and, as such, fell within the definition. Section 79(7) defines premises as including land. Reliance was placed on a passage from the speech of Viscount Dilhorne in *Maunsell v Olins* [1975] AC 373, [1975] 1 All ER 16, but that case was concerned with the word premises in a different context, namely that of the law of landlord and tenant.

It was argued that premises included structures of one kind or another and that that approach is supported by a provision in the Interpretation Act 1978. Section 5 of the 1978 Act states that "Land includes buildings and other structures, land covered with water, and any estate, interest, easement, servitude, or right in or over land". Thus, the sewer in this case, being made of pipes laid under the ground, was, and is, a structure. Land includes a structure. Premises include land and therefore s.79(1)(a) applies to a public sewer.

The authorities that drove the Deputy Stipendiary Magistrate to the conclusion that premises in this context did not include a public sewer were *R v Parlby* [1889] QB 520 and *Fulham Vestry v London County Council* [1897] 2 QB 76. *Parlby* was a case specifically concerned with the predecessor of s.79(1)(a), namely s.91.1 of the 1875 Act. Its significance lay at the heart of the present case, and much of the submissions related to the appropriate construction or interpretation of Parlby.

In the 1875 Act it said

The provisions of... (the Public Health Act, 1875), ss 91 to 96, for the abatement of certain nuisances, do not apply to a nuisance arising from sewage tanks and works constructed under s 27 by a local board of health, and a court of summary jurisdiction has, therefore, no power, on proof of a nuisance so caused, to make an order for the abatement of such nuisance under s 96.

Wills J in Parlby had said:

In our opinion the provisions we have stated have no application to sewage works constructed under the powers of s 27; we think the words of s 91 do not include them, and we think they were not meant to include them. It is clear that the expression premises in such a state as to be a nuisance has not the wide application claimed for it by the respondents, who say that it is answered by any premises on which a nuisance exists. If that were so the enumeration of, at all events, the several kinds of nuisance specified under heads 2,3,4 and 6 would be unnecessary; we do not attempt to define every class of case to which the first head applies, but we think it is confined to cases in which the premises themselves are decayed, dilapidated, dirty, or out of order, as, for instance, where houses have been inhabited by tenants whose habits and ways of life have rendered them filthy or impregnated with disease, or where foul matter has been allowed to soak into walls or floors, or where they are so dilapidated as to be a source of danger to life and limb.

It is a significant fact that under the second head the various receptacles for running or stagnant water which may be foul stop with drains, which, by the interpretation clause, are not sewers;...

Fulham Vestry v London County Council was not concerned with the 1875 Act but with s.2(1)(b) of the Public Health (London) Act 1891. That was a provision rather similar but not the same as s.91.2 of the 1875 Act.

Those two authorities were considered by the Divisional Court in *R v Epping (Waltham Abbey) Justices ex parte Burlinson* [1948] KB 79, [1947] 2 All ER 537. Lord Goddard, CJ, speaking of the case of *Parlby*, said

That case seems to me to decide no more than this, that a nuisance alleged to arise from the construction of a sewage system is not one of the statutory nuisances within the sections of the Public Health Act, and that is really the whole of the decision in that case. No doubt there was an offensive smell arising from it, but the court would not hold that main sewers and sewage works of that description fell within the words of the section; they would not hold that it was one of these statutory nuisances in respect of which alone the justices had power to make an abatement order, and they said the case must be decided by the High Court.

It was *Parlby* and *Fulham Vestry* that caused the Deputy Stipendiary Magistrate to decide as he did. *Ex. p. Burlinson* was also cited. He therefore took them as representing a statement of the current law.

One submission for the local authority was that *Parlby* itself did not decide whether or not a public sewer is, or is not, a premises within the meaning of the section but merely drew a distinction between premises in such a state as to be a nuisance and premises on which a nuisance exists.

The second area of substantial dispute was whether the interpretation given to the word premises when the 1875 Act was the current legislation now applies, several Acts on, to the same word in s.79(1)(a) of the 1990 Act.

On behalf of the Respondent, it was submitted that it did, as illustrated by *Sterling Homes v Birmingham City Council* [1996] EnvLR 121. The issue there was whether another judicial decision under the 1875 Act, the case of *R v Wheatley* (1885) 16 QBD 34, which construed a provision in the 1875 Act, namely s.94, bound a Court in 1995 when construing a substantially similar provision in the 1990 Act. It was concluded that the 1990 Act was not a merely consolidating measure, and there was good practical reason for suggesting that Parliament did not in 1990 intend that such a specification was essential.

In that judgement, it was said that the similarity of wording suggested that, if the local authority decides to require works to be executed or other steps to be taken to abate the nuisance, Parliament intended the interpretation that the courts had put on substantially the same provisions in the Act of 1875 (which had been repeated in the Act of 1936) to be perpetuated. Had Parliament intended to repeat the pattern of s.58(1)(b) of the 1974 Act, it would have followed the wording of that subsection. It was concluded that such works and other steps as are required by an abatement notice issued under s.80(1) of the 1990 Act must specify the works or the other steps, as was decided in R v Wheatley.

The decision in The *East Riding of Yorkshire* case also referred to Halsbury's Statutes, Fourth Edition, Volume 35, and the annotation to s.79 says "Premises. Sewage, disposal works, and public sewers are not included in this term: *R v Parlby* cf *Fulham Vestry v LCC*".

It was concluded that *Parlby* was applicable as the appropriate construction of s.79(1)(a) is correct. And it was concluded that Parliament, in 1990, intended to incorporate the existing jurisprudence in relation to the same and similar wording under the 1875 and subsequent Acts. If there had been an intention to depart from the existing jurisprudence, it would have been expressly stated in the 1990 Act.

The fact that there is a significant difference between the 1875 Act and the 1990 Act in that, for example, a new and more developed appeal procedure in relation to abatement notices was held not to have any bearing upon the case.

It was therefore concluded that the word premises in s.79(1)(a) does not include a public sewer. That decision only related to whether or not there was a statutory nuisance and was not concerned, in any way, with any liability at common law or any remedy in private law that may accrue to any particular landowner.

Hounslow London Borough Council v Thames Water Utilities Ltd
[2003] EWHC 1197 (Admin) [2003] All ER (D) 347 (May)

In July 2001, LB Hounslow served an abatement notice on Thames Water under s.80 of the EPA'90. The notice specified that an odour amounting to a nuisance had occurred and was likely to recur at premises known as Mogden Sewage Treatment Works, for which the company was responsible. The company appealed against the notice to the Magistrates' Court. A preliminary hearing was held to determine whether the sewage works constituted premises within the meaning of s.79(1)(d) of the 1990 Act. Section 79 defines, subject to exceptions, statutory nuisances as including

(1)(a) any premises in such a state as to be prejudicial to health or a nuisance; ... (d) any dust, steam, smell or other effluvia arising on industrial, trade or business premises and being prejudicial to health or a nuisance ... (7) ... premises are used for industrial purposes where they are used for the purposes of any treatment or process ...

The district judge quashed the notice. He was of the opinion that sewage works were excluded from the operation of s.79(1)(d), having relied on authority from 1889. That case construed the predecessor section to s.79(1)(a) and held that the term 'premises' was not apt to embrace sewage works.

The local authority then appealed by way of case stated. The Divisional Court was of the opinion that, on their true construction, sewage works were not excluded from the operation of s.79(1)(d) of the 1990 Act. The Respondent's case was that s.79 did not apply to sewage treatment works because of *R v Parlby and others* [1889] 22 QB. 520 (decision under the 1875 Act, which was a predecessor of Section 79(1)(a) of the 1990 Act). The Divisional Court was told that there had been no subsequent decision directly upon the proper construction of Section 79(1)(d) or its predecessors. It was held that it was possible to distinguish the history behind s.79(1)(a) from that of the provisions in s.79(1)(d). In general, s.79(1) was inclusive subject to identified exceptions and when framing s.79(1)(d), Parliament had not intended to exclude any particular premises, including land, from its operation unless by necessary implication or the exclusion was identified in the subsections. Although the 1889 (*Parlby*) construction of the words 'premises' was still applicable to s.79(1)(a), it was not possible to transplant that construction to the use of the same word in s.79(1)(d) when, by s.79(7), premises were deemed to be 'used for industrial purposes where they were used for the purposes of any treatment or process', and the definition of statutory nuisance by identification of conditions had been completely recast by the 1990 Act as Parliament's intention had been to restate the law.

On further application to quash the abatement notice in September 2004, the judgement in November 2004 decided that the best practicable means had not been employed despite substantial expenditure and that the statutory nuisance continued. No reason was found to uphold the appeal except that insufficient time (60 days) had been given. This was not seen as sufficient to quash the notice, and the terms of the notice were varied by substituting two years from the date of the decision for completion of the work to abate the statutory nuisance.

Note: LB Bexley successfully defended an appeal in the Crown Court by Thames Water against an abatement notice served on the company as the result of odours from the Crossness Sewage Works. It was held that the company had not done all it could to prevent odour nuisance (see ENDS Report 364 May 2005).

Dobson and another v Thames Water Utilities and another
[2009] All ER (D) 252 (Jan)

The essence of the claimants' claim was that odours and mosquitoes from the works had caused a private nuisance as a result of the negligence of the sewerage undertaker in the way they operated the Mogden sewage treatment works. It was claimed that the defendant had breached their rights to respect for private and family life and protection of property under the art 8 of the European Convention on Human Rights. The claimants were divided between claimants who occupied properties as owners or lessees and those who occupied properties without any legal interest in them. The principal points for determination were (i) the proper basis for an award of common law damages for a transitory nuisance where no lasting damage to the claimant's land or loss of capital value had been occasioned; (ii) whether such an award included damages recovered by the property owner or owners on behalf of any non-property owner member of the same household; (iii) the proper basis for an award of damages for infringement of Article 8 rights in such a case of transitory nuisance; and (iv) the effect, if any, which an award of common law damages under (i) had upon the decision as to the proper remedy to be awarded in respect of the same acts to a non-property owning member of the same household who brought a claim for infringement of art 8.

The appeal by Thames from the High Court decision was allowed in part. Under the HRA 1998, damages should not be the main remedy, but the courts reserve the right to award modest compensatory damages. The Court of Appeal concluded it was not possible to state as a question of law that claimants such as children should be excluded from taking action because their parents had secured damages based on diminution of value under a nuisance claim (that would require a proprietary interest in the land affected). Each case must be considered on its merits, but barring unusual circumstances, a court would be reluctant to award substantial damages under the HRA to children whose parents had already received damages under a nuisance claim.

This decision is part of the first stage in examining preliminary issues of law before a full action is heard, and the appeal by Thames was against the decision of the High Court (Technology and Construction Court) to allow claims by individuals even where they did not have a legal interest in the affected property. More than 1,000 residents are parties to a group action that has secured funding from the Legal Services Commission as a result of the smells from the Mogden treatment works and who became frustrated at the slow pace of action using statutory nuisance.

R (on the application of Thames Water Utilities Ltd) v Bromley Magistrates' Court [2008] All ER (D) 352 (Jul) [2008] EWHC 1763 (QB) and [2013] EWHC 472 (Admin)

The claimant statutory undertaker was prosecuted by the Environment Agency under s.33 of the Environmental Protection Act 1990 for depositing controlled waste on land without a waste management licence.

A preliminary issue was raised by the claimant as to whether, as a matter of law, sewage escaping from pipes maintained by a statutory undertaker was 'controlled waste'. The district judge determined that he had no jurisdiction to determine that issue, and the claimant applied for judicial review. The Divisional Court decided (see [2005] All ER (D) 265 (May)) that the district judge had had jurisdiction to decide the issue. Rather than remitting the matter, however, it was decided that a reference would be made to the European Court of Justice.

The question referred was whether sewage that escaped from a sewage network maintained by a statutory sewage undertaker pursuant to the Urban Waste Water Treatment Directive (EEC) 91/271 (the UWWTD) and/or the WIA'91 amounted to 'directive waste' for the purposes of the Waste Framework Directive (Directive (EEC) 75/442) (the WFD), and if the answer was in the affirmative, whether the aforesaid sewage was excluded from the scope of 'directive waste' by virtue of art 2(1)(b)(iv) of the WFD, in particular, by virtue of the UWWTD and/or the WIA'91.

The European Court of Justice (ECJ) decided that the UWWTD was not 'other legislation' within the meaning of article 2(1)(b) of the WFD, so it fell to the national court to ascertain whether national rules might be regarded as being 'other legislation' within the meaning of that provision. They ruled that that would be the case if those national rules contained precise provisions organising the management of the waste in question and if they were such as to ensure a level of protection of the environment equivalent to that guaranteed by the WFD. Following that judgement, the matter was returned to the Divisional Court for it to determine the preliminary issue in light of the answers given by the European Court of Justice.

The court ruled that Sewage escaping from pipes maintained by a statutory undertaker was 'controlled waste' within the meaning of Section 33 of the 1990 Act.

There were no 'precise provisions' governing the management of waste that escaped unintentionally from the sewerage system. Accordingly, they were not 'covered by other legislation' in the sense explained by the European Court of Justice. That was not surprising, since escapes were by definition unplanned and therefore outside the scope of the ordinary management regime. However, that was no reason for them not to be subject to the criminal sanctions otherwise thought appropriate for the deposit of controlled waste. There was nothing unfair about that.

In this particular case, if the claimant could show that it had taken all reasonable precautions and exercised all due diligence (exercised the Duty of Care under s.34), it would have a defence.

Subsequent Judicial Review considered the question of whether an unintentional escape from a sewage system constituted a 'deposit' of controlled waste for the purposes of Section 33(1)(a) EPA 1990. It was no longer disputed, following the ECJ ruling, that the substance was controlled waste. It was held in the Magistrates' Court that there was indeed a deposit, and that the due diligence defence in section 33(7)(a) did not apply, leading to Thames' conviction as it was concluded that the unintended escape of sewage amounted to a 'deposit' within s.33(1)(a) of the Act.

United Utilities Water plc v Moss Rose Piggeries Ltd *[2006] All ER (D) 338 (Jun)*

The defendant company operated a pig farm. It was charged with discharging trade effluent into the public sewer without consent or authorisation, contrary to s.118(5) of the WIA'91. Before the deputy district judge, the defendant accepted that the discharges had been made but argued that they had in fact been authorised by an oral agreement with the prosecution's predecessor. The prosecution argued, inter alia, that any such agreement had been terminated by a letter giving the defendant three months' notice to that effect. The deputy district judge found, inter alia, that there was an agreement between the parties and that that agreement had not been terminated because three months' notice was unreasonable. He expressly declined to make detailed findings as to the terms of the agreement. The prosecution appealed by way of case stated. Meanwhile, it had issued a letter giving 12 months' notice of its intention to determine any agreement.

Having regard to the questions asked, issues arose, *inter alia*, as to whether the decision that three months' notice was not reasonable was one that a reasonable tribunal could have made and whether the defendant had the evidential burden to establish the existence of an agreement, and, having done so, was it for the prosecution to prove that the discharges were not in accordance with the agreement. The prosecution also complained of the failure to make detailed findings as to the terms of the agreement.

The appeal would be dismissed.

The defendant had the evidential burden of establishing the existence of an agreement, and having done so, it was for the prosecution to prove that the discharges were not in accordance with it.

In this case, the prosecution had not obtained from the deputy district judge the findings that would require a guilty verdict. An acquittal was justified based on the findings that had been made. Furthermore, it was not clear what kind of finding as to the terms of the agreement could touch on the question of adequate notice.

Although the district judge had failed to make detailed findings as to the terms of the agreement, having regard to the fresh notice to terminate that had been given and to the prosecution's concern to stop the discharge, the defendant's acquittal would, in all the circumstances, be affirmed.

Environment Agency v Biffa Waste Services Ltd and another
Queen's Bench Division (Divisional Court), March 2006

On or before 1 April 2003, a sewer belonging to Severn Trent Water Ltd (STW) became blocked. Consequently, polluting matter, such as sewage, was discharged into an adjacent stream that was controlled water for the purposes of s.85(1) of the Water Resources Act 1991. On 3 April, the sewerage undertaker informed the first defendant, Biffa Waste Services Ltd (Biffa), of the incident, and Biffa undertook to attend the site of the blockage with a jetting lorry and attempt to clear the blockage. On arrival, it became clear that jetting would not clear the blockage. Subsequently, STW informed the Environment Agency, which then attended the site. On arrival, the environment officer employed by the agency found a Biffa manager and two operatives at the site, along with an employee of STW who was actively involved and directing the operation.

STW then appointed a civil engineering contractor to clear the blockage. The plan formulated by the civil engineering contractor could not be carried out immediately, and therefore Biffa arranged for the second defendant, Eurotech Environmental Ltd (Eurotech), to commence 'tankering' so as to prevent sewage from discharging into the controlled waters pending clearance of the blockage. Eurotech was contracted to tanker until 6.30 am the next morning. There was no agreement to provide a relief tanker. When the tankering ceased, sewage was again discharged into the controlled waters.

On 4 April, the civil engineering contractor attended the site and cleared the blockage. STW pleaded guilty to an information that it had caused polluting matter, namely sewage, to enter controlled waters contrary to s.85(1) of the 1991 Act. On 7 April 2004, further information was laid by the agency, the prosecuting authority, against the first and second defendants, alleging that they had caused and/or knowingly permitted polluting matter to enter controlled waters contrary to ss 85(1) and (6) of the 1991 Act. On 24 May 2005, the district judge acquitted the first defendant of the charges on the ground that he was not satisfied to the criminal standard of proof that Biffa had any responsibility for the sewer on that day other than to provide such support and services, including tankering, as were required of it by STW, which it had done. The district judge also acquitted the second defendant of the charges. The prosecution appealed by way of case stated.

An issue arose, inter alia, as to whether Biffa had any responsibility for the sewer on 3 April other than to provide such support and services, including tinkering, as were required of it by STW, which it had done.

On the evidence, the district judge had been entitled to conclude that Biffa's responsibility for the sewer on that day was to provide such support and services as required by STW and to have acquitted her accordingly.

The Manchester Ship Canal Company Limited v United Utilities Water Ltd *in the Supreme Court*

The Court of Appeal gave judgement in this case [2021] EWHC 1571 (Ch) [2022] EWCA Civ 852 regarding potential avenues of redress in respect of discharges of sewage into waterbodies and found in favour of the WaSC.

The appeal formed part of a long-running dispute about discharges into the Manchester Ship Canal from sewers operated by United Utilities Water Ltd ("UU"). After the Canal Company threatened to bring a private law claim in nuisance and/or trespass against UU in respect of discharges of foul water, UU commenced a claim for a declaration, to the effect that no such cause of action was available to the Canal Company (in the absence of any allegation of negligence or deliberate wrongdoing). The essence of UU's argument was a contention that the proposed causes of action were impliedly ousted by the WIA 1991, which provides a statutory enforcement mechanism for breaches of duty by sewerage undertakers.

At first instance, the court had found in favour of UU. The Court of Appeal dismissed the Canal Company's appeal, essentially on the basis that the case was indistinguishable from *Marcic v Thames Water Utilities Ltd* [2003] UKHL 66, discussed previously. The Court of Appeal rejected the Canal Company's argument that it was a material point of distinction that the present case concerned discharges of sewage into a waterbody rather than escapes of sewage onto land, notwithstanding the terms of some provisions in WIA' 91 (notably s.117(5)-(6)) that appeared to preserve the ability to advance private law claims flowing from the discharge of foul water into waterbodies. Such provisions had not been considered in *Marcic*.

The Court of Appeal also considered an appeal (in separate proceedings between the Canal Company and UU) in relation to sewage outfalls that had originally been permitted by way of agreements that were, on their face, terminable by the Canal Company. Again, it was held that UU had a continued statutory right to drain through such outfalls, notwithstanding the Canal Company's termination or purported termination of the agreements. The Court of Appeal allowed the Canal Company's appeal on this issue.

The essence of UU's argument has always been that private law claims were impliedly ousted by WIA' 91, which provides a statutory enforcement mechanism for breaches of duty by sewerage undertakers. While UU was successful before both the High Court and the Court of Appeal. The Canal Company appealed to the Supreme Court, the issue being: can The Manchester Ship Canal Company Limited bring a private law claim in nuisance and/or trespass against UU in respect of unauthorised discharges of untreated foul water by UU into the canal? At the time of writing, judgement is still awaited.

Notes

1 *Fish Legal v Information Commissioner* [2015] UKUT 0052 (AAC).
2 Scottish Water was formed in 2002 by the merger of the West, East and North Water Authorities and is a statutory corporation providing water and sewerage services in Scotland and accountable to the Scottish Government.
3 https://en.wikipedia.org/wiki/Water_privatisation_in_England_and_Wales#cite_note-plimmer-19
4 See: https://www.theguardian.com/environment/2022/nov/30/more-than-70-percent-english-water-industry-foreign-ownership
5 See https://www.theguardian.com/environment/2022/aug/19/water-firms-england-wales-litres-leaky-pipes-ofwat
6 See https://www.gov.uk/government/news/record-90m-fine-for-southern-water-following-ea-prosecution
7 See https://www.gov.uk/government/publications/water-and-sewerage-companies-in-england-environmental-performance-report-2021/water-and-sewerage-companies-in-england-environmental-performance-report-2021
8 https://publications.parliament.uk/pa/cm199798/cmselect/cmenvtra/266ii/et0202.htm
9 The EA lost an appeal against that decision see [2002] EWCA Civ 5.
10 Sewerage Sector Guidance – approved documents can be found on the Water UK website at https://www.water.org.uk/sewerage-sector-guidance-approved-documents/
11 The Water Industry (Schemes for Adoption of Private Sewers) Regulations 2011 Si 2011 No 1566 came into force on 1 July 2011 and ceased to have effect on 30 June 2018 and were made under sections 102(4) (as modified by section 105A(6)(a) of the WIA'91), 105A and 213(2)(f) of the WIA'91.
12 In this it said "access points and sewers should be sited where reasonable access and visibility can be gained by the sewerage undertaker. They should avoid rear gardens or enclosed locations" https://assets.publishing.service.gov.uk/government/uploads/system/uploads/attachment_data/file/82516/new-build-sewers-consult-annexb-sos-standards-111220.pdf
13 s.21 as amended.
14 30.48 metres.
15 SI 1989 No 1156; SI 1990 No 1629; and SI 1992 No 339.
16 https://assets.publishing.service.gov.uk/government/uploads/system/uploads/attachment_data/file/1128073/The_review_for_implementation_of_Schedule_3_to_The_Flood_and_Water_Management_Act_2010.pdf

17 See https://assets.publishing.service.gov.uk/government/uploads/system/up-loads/attachment_data/file/415773/sustainable-drainage-technical-standards. pdf and also for Wales https://www.gov.wales/national-standards-sustainable-drainage-systems-suds

18 Environmental Permitting (England and Wales) Regulations 2016 SI 2016 No 1154 (These Regulations provide a consolidated system of environmental permitting in England and Wales. They replace the Environmental Permitting (England and Wales) Regulations 2010 SI 2010 No 675.

19 See *Anglian Water Services Ltd v R* [2003] EWCA Crim 2243 ([2003] EWCA Crim 2243, [2004] 1 Cr App R (S) 62, [2004] 1 Cr App Rep (S) 62, [2004] Env LR 10, [2004] JPL.

20 *Hounslow London Borough Council v Thames Water Utilities Ltd* [2003] EWHC 1197 (Admin) [2003].

21 as amended by the Building (Amendment) Regulations 2001, SI 2001/3335, reg 3(4)(a).

22 Drainage is defined in s.21(2) of the Act to include "the conveyance, by means of a sink and any other necessary appliance, of refuse water and the conveyance of rain-water from roofs".

23 Schedule 3 to the Flood and Water Management Act 2010 extends the power under this subsection to sustainable drainage systems as defined in regulations under that Schedule.

24 s.219(1),(2) of the WIA'91.

25 See: Housing Health and Safety Rating System – Operating Guidance (Guidance about inspections and assessment of hazards given under s.9 Housing Act 2004), ODPM, 2006 – but note the HHSRS is subject of a review in 2023.

26 *Marcic v Thames Water plc* [2003] UKHL 66.

27 https://www.bailii.org/ew/cases/EWHC/TCC/2017/460.html

References

1 Cavendish C, 2022, Privatising water was never going to work. *The Telegraph* 19 August 2022, https://www.ft.com/content/f752468a-5819e2-4928-9e3b-ee5bcce252aa

2 Hall D, 2022, *Water and sewerage company finances 2021: dividends and investment - and company attempts to hide dividends*, PSIRU University of Greenwich Working Paper Public Services International Research Unit (PSIRU), University of Greenwich.

3 Yearwood K, 2018, *The privatised water industry in the UK. An ATM for investors.* Public Services International Research Unit (PSIRU), University of Greenwich, https://gala.gre.ac.uk/id/eprint/21097/20/21097%20YEARWOOD_The_Privatised_Water_Industry_in_the_UK_2018.pdf

4 Ofwat, 2022, *Design and construction guidance for foul and surface water sewers offered for adoption under the code for adoption agreements for water and sewerage companies operating wholly or mainly in England*, Approved Version 2.2 can be accessed at https://www.water.org.uk/sewerage-sector-guidance-approved-documents/

4 Who makes sure legal obligations are met?

Operation of CSO.s and discharges to water

As we will see in the next chapter, the Government, particularly Defra, Ofwat, and the Environment Agencies, have a role, although it is the WaSCs that actually operate the CSO.s. In England, the Agency has been cut back to such an extent that it is argued the staff cannot do their jobs, so it is no longer a deterrent to polluters. Although it has a large budget, it is reported that this is not being directed towards protecting or improving the environment. Government grants to the agency rose from £880 million to £1.05 billion between 2020 and 2022, and money for flood operations has steadily increased, but funding for environmental protection work has slumped from about £170 million in 2009–10 to a low of £76 million in 2019–20 and £94 million in 2021,[1] and funding for this work was halved in the ten years to 2022.

In fact, it is campaigners such as Surfers Against Sewage and Feargal Sharkey, as well as local groups and activists who have highlighted the issue.

The Environmental Agencies regulate intermittent discharges from sewer overflows and wastewater treatment works (WWTW) through environmental permits. These permits require the WaSCs to construct and maintain sewerage systems according to their best technical knowledge not entailing excessive cost. As part of this, the WaSCs are supposed to identify storm overflows that need improvement.

The Environment Agency argues that it works closely with the WaSCs to ensure that they are closely monitoring and reporting back on their discharge activity. These data are supposed to help provide an understanding of where the system is not operating as it should so that water companies can target investigations and investments. However, it has been argued that the Environment Agency is failing to detect thousands of illegal spills because it is not scrutinising the available data closely enough.

Yet the EA successfully brought only our water company prosecutions in 2019, resulting in a total of £1,297,000 in fines. Some fines do grab the headlines, but the number of actions seems small by comparison with the scale of the problem. For example, in April 2023, South West Water was fined more

DOI: 10.1201/9781003375647-4

than £2.1 million after admitting causing pollution of controlled waters in Devon and Cornwall. It admitted six offences of illegal discharge activities and seven offences of contravening environmental permit conditions. As another example, Anglian Water pleaded guilty and was fined £2.65 million after allowing untreated sewage to overflow into the North Sea following prosecution by the Environment Agency. A catalogue of failures by the company to manage and monitor effluent at a Water Recycling Centre in Essex led to sewage being discharged into the sea because the WaSC decommissioned a piece of equipment, which led to the conditions for untreated sewage to be released into the North Sea. To put these fines into perspective, in 2022, the revenues of Thames Water were £2,176.9 million (the largest), Anglian Water was £1,299.7 million, South West Water was £584.6 million, and Southern Water was £823.5 million.[2]

In Event Duration Monitoring, the EA requires water and sewerage companies to measure how often and for how long, storm overflows are used. The number of overflows monitored across the network has increased from 800 in 2016 to more than 12,700 in 2021, the equivalent of almost nine in ten storm overflows.[3]

It is worth noting that when it came to assessing and classifying bathing waters affected by sewage pollution, the Environment Agency got it wrong so far as the regulations are concerned (*Anglian Water Service Ltd v Environment Agency* [2020] EWHC 3544 (Admin), [2021] All ER (D) 24 (Jan)) because it failed to take account of heavy rainfall that had increased the level of coliforms when the water was sampled and did not "disregard the samples on the basis that they had been taken during a 'short-term pollution' event".

Ofwat has a role too. In 2021–22, the EA and Ofwat launched Operation Standard, an investigation into potential widespread non-compliance by water and sewerage companies at WWTW.[4] In 2019, Ofwat introduced a package of allowances and incentives for the next five years, setting water companies the challenge of reducing pollution incidents by a third and also requiring them to invest £4.8 billion in environmental improvements. Ofwat also has the power to issue fines up to 10% of a company's turnover for the affected business and order companies to take the action necessary to return to compliance where they are in breach.

The Office for Environmental Protection has an important role in holding the government to account. In June 2022, it announced that it was to carry out an investigation into the roles of Ofwat, the Environment Agency, and the Defra Secretary of State in the regulation of combined sewer overflows (CSO.s) in England. The aims of the investigation are to determine whether these authorities have failed to comply with their respective duties in relation to the regulation, including the monitoring and enforcement, of water companies' own duties to manage sewage. In doing so, we will seek to clarify the respective duties. The investigation follows a complaint submitted to the Interim

Office for Environmental Protection OEP by Salmon & Trout Conservation UK, further illustrating the role of campaigning and environmental groups.

In its report "Tak*ing stock: protecting, restoring and improving the environment in England*" [1], the OEP says that water pollution from agricultural runoff, discharges from sewage treatment works, and combined sewer overflows are significant pressures in freshwater and coastal environments. Whilst overflow discharges are increasingly well documented and have an acute impact on the environment, treated sewage has a chronic impact, despite the improvements in treatment over the years. This limits long-term improvements in aquatic ecosystems.

In a 2023 report, the OEP records research that found that the UK Government has not consistently completed legally required Post-Implementation Reviews of environmental laws [2]. Regulation 12A of the Urban Wastewater Treatment (England and Wales) Regulations 1994 (under which the appropriate authority must prepare and publish a situation report on the disposal of urban wastewater and sludge, review and assess compliance with these Regulations in each agglomeration, and prepare and publish a report) was actually published, albeit belatedly.

The House of Commons Environmental Audit Committee 2022 report on water quality in rivers highlighted the problems and brought further pressure on the Government [3]. Quoting evidence for Surfers Against Sewage that poor water quality was a public health issue, "putting water users at risk of exposure to harmful viruses and antimicrobial-resistant bacteria causing sickness, distress, and in some cases, long-term health effects". The report highlighted that there "was no monitoring in river environments in the way that we do on the coast because there is not a legal obligation to do that in the same way' if they are not designated bathing waters. There was also evidence that sewage treatment works and the rivers they discharge into were becoming breeding grounds for antimicrobial resistance. A study of UK coastal waters found that 11 of the 97 waters sampled contained *E. coli* resistant to antibiotics".

Campaigning groups and NGOs, more than anyone else as we have seen, have highlighted the condition of our waters as the result of the excessive operation of the CSO.s. Surfers Against Sewage even has an App for tracking real-time sewage discharge and pollution risks around the UK.[5]

Sewer flooding of properties

The primary regulator is Ofwat. Section 94 of the Water Industry Act 1991 (WIA91) places a duty on sewerage companies, amongst other things, to maintain their sewers to ensure that their area is effactually drained. The Director must take enforcement action under Section 18(1) WIA91 where satisfied that a company is, or is likely to be, in breach of its Section 94 duty. Under s.19(1) WIA91, there are three exceptions to the duty to take enforcement action. In summary, these are cases where the breach of duty is not serious, where the company has given the Director an undertaking to take whatever action the Director considers appropriate, for example, to carry out remedial works, and where the Director cannot take enforcement action because this would be incompatible with certain of his other duties.

Ofwat will consider each case on its own facts. In terms of sewer flooding, the factors that we are likely to consider when assessing whether the company is in breach include the following:

- Physical factors relevant to the flooding, for example, the location of the property
- The severity of the weather at the time of flooding – factors outside the company's control that are contributing to the flooding. These could include inadequate drainage arrangements for which the company is not responsible, for example, highway, surface, or land drainage – where flooding has resulted from a blockage, the cause of the blockage (e.g. third-party action and a lack of maintenance)
- The number of properties affected
- The frequency and extent of the flooding
- Whether the flooding is internal (inside the building) or external (e.g. restricted to gardens or outbuildings) – usage of the property – for example, whether it is domestic or non-domestic
- Whether the company has a scheme of work reasonably prioritised

Ofwat has issued guidance[6] to enable all companies to report on sewer flooding for the defined year at a reasonable level of accuracy and with a common approach. Reporting of flooding incidents is supposed to be done in accordance with each company's quality assurance process.

This guidance covers two measures of flooding incidents, and both should include flooding due to overloading of the sewers (lack of hydraulic capacity) and other causes. The two measures are

1   The number of internal flooding incidents per year
2   The number of external flooding incidents per year

For both measures, this guidance covers how companies can report the number of incidents, both including and excluding the impact of severe weather.

A flooding incident is defined as the number of properties (or curtilages) flooded during each flooding event from a sewer that is the WaSC's responsibility. For example, 15 properties that suffered two flooding events during a year would count as 30 incidents. The guidance defines a flooding event as the escape of water from a sewerage system, irrespective of size, as evidenced by standing water, running water, or visible deposits of silt or sewage solids. The definitions of Internal and external flooding in this guidance are given in Chapter 1.

WaSCs are expected to "make all reasonable efforts to determine the number of properties affected by flooding". This seems like an obvious thing that they should do given the trauma that householders will suffer. As we have seen, flooding premises would make them "prejudicial to health" and therefore a statutory nuisance, at least in theory. If the WaSC acts promptly and improves the hydraulic capacity of the sewer, then there might be no reason for the local authority to take action, but what if they don't and properties suffer regular flooding from sewers?

WaSCs are expected to make site visits to the affected property and all neighbouring properties that may have been affected, taking into account factors such as topography and the proximity of adjacent properties.

CC Water has said that if a customer gets in touch about internal sewer flooding, WaSCs should respond within two hours, with a similar four-hour target for external flooding. Companies should also be proactive, for example, by anticipating where flooding might occur during bad weather. To understand people's experiences of sewer flooding, either inside or outside of the home, Consumer Council for Water (CCW) and Ofwat commissioned this qualitative research, published in 2022. For those who experience sewer flooding inside or outside of their homes, the response by wastewater companies often makes this experience even worse. This was a consistent finding among participants across England and Wales [4].

Table 4.1 Number of sewer flooding incidents in 2020–21 per 10,000 properties[a]

	Internal sewer flooding incidents	External sewer flooding incidents
Anglian Water	1.33	12.72
Dyr Cymru	2.05	25.82
Hafren Dyfrdwy[b]	2.81	
Northumbrian Water	1.89	29.95
Severn Trent Water	1.86	8.61
South West water	1.34	19.49
Southern Water	1.96	21.94
Thames Water	2.31	
United Utilities	4.47	20.11
Wessex Water	1.41	19.35
Yorkshire Water	3.34	21.63

Source: Ofwat.

[a]   https://www.ofwat.gov.uk/wp-content/uploads/2022/05/customer-experiences-of-sewer-flooding-a-joint-report-by-ccw-and-ofwat.pdf
[b]   Hafren Dyfrdwy is a company that provides water and wastewater treatment services operating in north east Wales, its wastewater services are in northern Powys.

If drains that are not the responsibility of the WaSCs discharge so as to cause a statutory nuisance or are otherwise inadequate, then again, local authorities can use the statutory nuisance provisions in the Environmental Protection Act 1990 to secure a remedy (equally, if it leads to ditches or watercourses becoming prejudicial to health or a nuisance, then s.259 of the Public Health Act 1936 is potentially available). The provisions of the Building Act 1984, as discussed previously (s.59), provide a remedy for unsatisfactory drains and private sewers.

It is unlikely that local authority EHPs will be aware of leaking drains, but one symptom of defective drainage is the presence of rats. There is a link between surface rat infestation and broken drainage, so it is worthwhile to check the drains where there are reports of rats on the surface and there are no other obvious environmental sources or possible harbourage. Local authorities can use either statutory nuisance powers or those in the Prevention of Damage by Pests Act 1949 (and the Building Act 1984) both to investigate and secure a remedy. Local authority EHPs should also remember that there is a potential to use statutory nuisance provisions where premises are put into such a state as to be prejudicial to health as the result of sewer flooding and action can be taken by the person responsible (the person to whose act, default, or sufferance the nuisance is attributable) – the WaSC.

Sewage on beaches, in coastal waters, and rivers

This is primarily the responsibility of the environmental agencies to make sure that discharges do not breach permit conditions, including those from CSOs. It remains a question whether the conditions attached to permits are sufficiently strict – if there is frequent pollution yet conditions are complied with, then it would seem not, certainly in the public's view.

As we have seen in the *exp Shelley* case again, it is possible for the local authority to use the statutory nuisance provisions, but there has to be an accumulation.

Discharges to sewers

Controlling what goes into the sewerage system is primarily the responsibility of the WaSCs, and it is in their interests to ensure that nothing enters the sewers that compromises the workings of the WWTW. The WaSCs have ultimate responsibility for what goes into the sewers for which they have responsibility. However "it can be difficult to control "fly-tipping' into sewers"

As we have seen, the WIA '91 gives the WaSCs powers to control discharges into its sewers, but how well they do this is open to question despite it being in their own interests. The water industry has had problems in the past identifying all the historic trade effluent discharges, as records appear to have been incomplete as a result of responsibilities changing over the decades since controls were first introduced. The problem for WaSCs is also polluting matter entering the sewers via manholes, i.e., fly-tipping into manholes.

For prescribed processes, both the WasC and environmental agencies have a role, as we have seen in Chapter 3.

Leaking and blocked sewerage

For public sewers that are the responsibility of the WaSCs, it seems that this is a matter for the companies themselves and the Capitalise Environment Agency, although it seems the latter is rarely involved even where it leads to pollution of groundwater.

For drains other than public laterals, this is a matter for local authorities at the district level, who have at their disposal a range of powers, as has been shown in Chapter 3. The problem is that for many local authorities, they lack the resources to investigate, and in reality, where a drain or sewer is blocked, that is not the responsibility of the WaSC, the owners of the property(ies) affected are likely to call in their own contractor. The problem is that not all contractors are adequately trained or knowledgeable and may not have any knowledge of the WRc Drain and Sewer Cleaning Manual [5]. This is a best practice guidance document covering both blockage clearance and planned sewer cleaning. This supersedes WRc's Sewer Jetting Code of Practice, with an extended scope to cover all commonly used methods of drain and sewer blockage clearance and cleaning. It should be noted that poorly executed clearing methods, such as excessive high-pressure jetting, can damage some materials and increase the risk of drains or sewers leaking.

Misconnections

In the previous chapter, we saw the legal provisions on connecting to a sewer that are the responsibility of the WaSC. This might be taken to mean there cannot be misconnections; that would be wrong. It is not impossible for contractors to make connections to sewers without the knowledge of the WaSC; this is entirely possible where the public sewer is one that was private until the transfer in 2011. The WaSC now has responsibility for correcting any misconnections to their public sewers or public laterals, although it is likely that they will only become aware of these when the defect becomes obvious.

The potential consequences of a misconnection that is left unaddressed can be disastrous for the environment, public health, and wildlife. According to Defra, there are still an estimated 150,000 to 500,000 homes with some sort of drain misconnection.[7]

For misconnections near houses, the local authority has powers already discussed under the Building Act 1984. Where, for example, a washing machine or other wastewater is connected to a surface water drain that discharges to a water course or soakaway, this would fall within the scope of Section 59 of the 1984 Act. That would be the case should such wastes be discharged to a surface water sewer that is the responsibility of the WaSC. At their worst, additional toilets have been misconnected to surface water drains and sewers. It is estimated that 15% of rivers in England and Wales have caused the waters to fail quality standards as a result of misconnections.

Where such a misconnection leads to pollution of controlled water, even from domestic premises, then the relevant Environment Agency could take action. It is an offence to cause or knowingly permit a water pollution discharge activity, that is, to pollute a controlled water, remembering that groundwater is included as a controlled water (although it is unlikely that action has ever been taken for pollution as the result of exfiltration). For England and Wales, the principal water pollution offences are contained in the Environmental Permitting (England and Wales) Regulations 2010,[8] so it is an offence to cause a discharge to water other than in accordance with a permit.

It is a strict liability offence. This means that intention is not a pre-requisite to proving the offence. If pollution is due to a chain of events, a person may be regarded as having caused pollution even if someone else's actions immediately triggered the incident. Being aware of a polluting incident and refusing to take reasonable prevention steps is also an offence.

We can see that, merely on the topic of misconnections, different agencies can be involved, depending on the impact of the misconnection. With some justification, WaSCs have urged local authorities to be more proactive in dealing with misconnections.

How good are the agencies involved?

We will look at what is being done and what could be done in the next chapter, but having looked at who is responsible for addressing some of the problems, how could they have been so far? Comment is made almost daily on how the environmental regulators, particularly the Environment Agency, are failing to enforce the existing legislation adequately and highlighting the inadequacies of government policy in this area.

The National Audit Office has pointed out that the environment agency's enforcement activities cannot be cross-subsidised from charges that the agency makes for permits and licences. Instead, it allocates resources to enforcement from its grant-in-aid funding for environmental protection. It is, therefore, dependent on the government allocating sufficient funds. This grant-in-aid funding fell by 80% between 2010–11 and 2020–21. Furthermore, the amount of grant-in-aid that is ring-fenced for particular projects, including non-enforcement activity, has grown. The number of vacancies has fluctuated over the past six years, with vacancies as a percentage of total compliance and enforcement staff reaching a 10% high in 2019, falling to 2% in 2021, and increasing again to 6% in 2022.[9]

In November 2022, the EA said that in the previous seven years it had brought 56 prosecutions of WaSCs, securing £141 million in fines.[10] It pointed out the two successful prosecutions of Anglian Water in October 2022 and that in 2022, eight successful prosecutions were brought by the EA, resulting in fines of over £3.6 million. For all that, the WaSCs do not appear to be acting quickly enough.

Unfortunately, there is no data on how well or frequently local authorities use their powers to resolve sewerage problems. Although local authorities might have information on their websites, there is no record of how frequently their powers are used. This is the type of information that used to be collected by the CIEH for the annual environmental health report, but that has not been done for many years. Perhaps, given the concerns about the relatively low profile of environmental health, this is something that should be resurrected.

Despite the government not providing sufficient resources and high-profile prosecutions of WaSCs, it can be argued that the approach to dealing with sewage pollution has been typified by a lack of effective enforcement. Is this because of a failure to recognise a public health issue?

Defra is responsible for sponsoring legislation and ensuring the EA is adequately resourced. The response to the CSO issue will be addressed in the next chapter, but as can be seen from the publicity surrounding sewage pollution, Defra's overall approach has been inadequate, to put it politely. This may also be a reflection of a government that is reluctant to tighten regulations.

Ofwat has always been concerned with sewer flooding incidents but has been weak on making the WaSCs invest more in the sewerage infrastructure and renewal of sewers to ensure adequate hydraulic capacity. It is relatively recently that it seems to have become more interested in the frequent operation of CSO.s. It argues that investment in the industry has roughly doubled since privatisation in 1989 and capital expenditure has been between £5 billion and £6 billion a year; the question is whether this is enough or has been well spent. Ofwat admits that in the 2015–20 period, water and sewerage companies actually underspent by 5% the price review allowances for investment in their wastewater facilities.[11]

The Office of Environmental Protection is relatively new, so it is perhaps too early to make any judgement, but at least initially, it would seem that it is taking its responsibilities seriously; whether the Government takes any notice is another question.

Already mentioned are Parliamentary Committees, and in particular the House of Commons Environmental Audit Committee, which has highlighted the problems for rivers and made a number of recommendations. In 2023, the Environment, Food, and Rural Affairs Committee launched a one-off inquiry into the Environment Agency and took oral evidence from the Chairman and Chief Executive, but as a Committee, it looks at all the work of Defra and has not given much, if any, time to this area of work.

As has already been made clear in other parts of this book, campaigning groups and NGOs have been very effective in highlighting the inadequacies of current controls, particularly when it comes to the operation of CSO.s. The next chapter includes more information about some of the campaigns and their implications for the future.

Notes

1 https://www.theguardian.com/environment/2022/jan/20/environment-agency-cuts-staff-blow-whistle
2 https://www.statista.com/statistics/1179995/leading-water-and-sewer-utilities-companies-in-the-united-kingdom/
3 https://environment.data.gov.uk/dataset/21e15f12-0df8-4bfc-b763-45226c16a8ac
4 https://assets.publishing.service.gov.uk/government/uploads/system/uploads/attachment_data/file/1115122/EA-Annual-Report-2021-22.pdf
5 https://www.sas.org.uk/water-quality/sewage-pollution-alerts/
6 https://www.ofwat.gov.uk/wp-content/uploads/2018/03/Reporting-guidance-sewer-flooding-updated-April-2018.pdf
7 https://www.ciwem.org/news/drain-misconnections
8 Regulations 38(1) and 12(1).
9 https://www.nao.org.uk/wp-content/uploads/2022/05/Environmental-compliance-and-enforcement.pdf
10 https://environmentagency.blog.gov.uk/2022/11/18/update-on-environment-agency-investigation-2/
11 https://www.ofwat.gov.uk/investment-in-the-water-industry/#qu1

References

1 OEP, 2022, *Taking stock: protecting, restoring and improving the environment in England*, OGL, Worcester, https://www.theoep.org.uk/node/381
2 OEP, 2023, *Post-Implementation Review of Environmental Law*, OGL, Worcester, https://www.theoep.org.uk/report/government-consistently-failing-complete-post-implementation-reviews-environmental-laws
3 House of Commons Environmental Audit Committee, 2022, Fourth Report of Session 2021–22 "Water Quality in Rivers", HC74.
4 Ofwat, 2022, *Customer experiences of sewer flooding: a joint report by CCW and Ofwat*, Crown copyright, available at https://www.ofwat.gov.uk/wp-content/uploads/2022/05/customer-experiences-of-sewer-flooding-a-joint-report-by-ccw-and-ofwat.pdf
5 WRc, 2020, *Manual of drain and sewer cleaning*, Helsby, Cheshire, https://wrc-knowledgestore.co.uk/products/drain-and-sewer-cleaning-manual

5 The future – what more is being, or can be done?

The principal public health responsibility for ensuring human faeces and viable human faecal bacteria, viruses, and other pollutants do not get into waterways people might use recreationally rests with the water companies and their directors. These same players are responsible for ensuring that there is no environmental harm as a result of their activities.

The Government and regulators are responsible for setting the standards and the performance criteria. Whether these are adequate is a moot point. In this chapter, I look at what is being done and what can be done in the future, including campaigns.

Combined Sewer Overflows (CSOs) are used to protect the works under peak dry weather flow conditions. Such frequent, and in some cases independent of rainfall, use of CSO.s could have detrimental effects on the receiving environment as well as put thousands of water users at risk. The findings of research using CSO monitoring data inform policymakers about the causes of the problem and should help the industry demonstrate the need for capital investment in infrastructure. The problem has been a lack of investment, or at least inadequate investment, over the years, despite the intentions of privatisation, and the infrastructure is often taken for granted, yet it is critical to our future prosperity. Unfortunately, the importance of such infrastructure is only recognised when it is not functioning [1]. CSO.s are not something that Environmental Health Officers (Practitioners) can address directly, but there are ways that they can intervene to reduce the flow into combined sewers by acting to ensure near-house drainage is sound. They can also campaign, as this book has shown that discharges of sewage into waters increase the risks to public health.

As has been shown in Chapter 3, it is very difficult for private individuals or persons affected to take private legal action, so it is very much down to campaigns to get action to reduce the harmful impacts of sewage pollution on the environment and public health.

This chapter will focus on the steps that the WaSCs and the Government can or are taking, as well as the practical steps that local authorities and Environmental Health Practitioners can take to reduce the risk of pollution. It will

DOI: 10.1201/9781003375647-5

also look at what has changed or is likely to change as a result of the Environment Act 2021 and what the Government and other agencies are doing and could do to reduce sewage escaping into the environment.

Central government

This section refers to the central government as a whole, for although Defra is the main government department with responsibility, other departments have an interest in the issue.

First and foremost, many will argue that the water industry should be renationalised. In truth, it was never "nationalised". The water industry grew out of local government and the Victorian recognition of the need to improve public health, with local government investing in sewerage and clean water (and keeping them separate). Whether "nationalisation" is the answer is moot, but what is required is greater government control, which must include directed investment. Thérèse Coffey, the Secretary of State, is reported as admitting "she cannot end the sewage scandal, in what critics are calling a "complete abdication of duty". She said "upgrading the sewage network to stop spills could add hundreds of pounds each to people's bills".[1] This then justifies the Government increasing controls over the companies in return for increased government investment for both the renewal of sewers and wastewater treatment as well as improved monitoring of CSO.s. The government has already conceded that it has made no assessment of the impact of dumping sewage pollution in shellfish waters. This is despite figures revealing more than 80,000 sewage spills took place in shellfish waters during the last three years.[2]

If Governments do not exist to protect public health, then what are they for? Yet Defra is not seen as a "public health" department. Indeed, the Department has been described as "dysfunctional"[3] "with ministers and officials divided on key areas of policy, including air and water pollution targets issued under the 2021 Environment Act". This is not helpful and perhaps explains in part why there seems to be a lack of leadership on this issue. After Brexit, Defra has the largest review exercise of any government department, and this seems to be putting pressure on departmental administration. This also follows on from years of cuts to the civil service. It is no wonder Defra is struggling to take action to set new pollution targets.

There are solutions to getting storm overflows back to only functioning in very high rainfall conditions, although with extreme weather as a result of global heating, this might still be more frequent than desirable. The Government has suggested that what is required is better operational management, innovation, and investment. This might be seen as the job of the WaSCs, but without pressure from Government, this is unlikely to progress as quickly as the public health imperative requires, as can be seen from the proposals put forward by the Government.

Government proposals

In Spring 2022, the government consulted on the Storm Overflows Discharge Reduction Plan. This consultation outlined proposed targets to guide the water industry in achieving progressive reductions in the frequency of discharges from storm overflows and the impact of such discharges on ecology and public health. The proposed targets focussed on:

- Eliminating impacts on ecology by 2050
- Reducing the frequency of discharges to bathing waters to meet Environment Agency spill limits by 2035
- Ensuring that overflows do not discharge above an average of ten rainfall events per year by 2050.

In theory, the Environment Act 2021 puts in place more protection against water pollution than ever before, including measures to deliver progressive reductions in the impacts of storm overflows on the environment and public health. There was a duty on the government to produce a statutory plan by 1 September 2022 to reduce discharges from storm overflows and their adverse impact, and to report to Parliament on progress.

The Storm Overflows Discharge Reduction Plan was published in August 2022 [2] and presented to Parliament as required under s.141(A)8 of the WIA'91 and s.84(3) of the Environment Act 2021 by the then Secretary of State. The plan sets new targets and is intended to require water companies to deliver an infrastructure programme to achieve these targets. The Government hoped that by 2025, water companies would have reduced overflow discharges from 2020 levels by around 25%.

The plan now is that:

- By 2035, water companies will have improved all overflows discharging into or near every designated bathing water and improved 75% of overflows discharging to high-priority sites.
- By 2050, no storm overflows will be permitted to operate outside of unusually heavy rainfall or to cause any adverse ecological harm.

The Government expects WaSCs to ensure their infrastructure keeps pace with increasing external pressures, such as urban growth and climate change, without these pressures leading to greater numbers of discharges.

The monitoring requirements on WaSCs have been "strengthened" to ensure a comprehensive picture of the use and impact of storm overflows. The duties in the Environment Act 2021 aim to ensure there is information on which WaSCs can be held to account by the Government and the regulators, who should take enforcement action where water companies are not meeting their legal obligations. This, of course, depends on the regulators having adequate resources to take action. The Environment Agency could take more enforcement action now, except that it has suffered from cuts to staffing as set out in the previous chapter.

The aim is that WaSCs will only be permitted to discharge from a storm overflow where they can demonstrate that there is no local adverse ecological impact. These proposals are now necessary because the Government and its MPs voted down amendments to the Environment Bill to Place a duty on sewerage undertakers to take all reasonable steps to ensure untreated sewage is not discharged from storm overflows and improve enforcement of illegal discharges.

The headline target must be achieved for most (at least 75%) of storm overflows discharging in or close to high priority sites by 2035 – this is still a long way off, only relates to priority sites, and illustrates that investment levels have not been sufficient since privatisation. High-priority sites are Sites of Special Scientific Interest (SSSIs), Special Areas of Conservation, Urban Wastewater Treatment Regulations sensitive areas, chalk streams, and waters currently failing ecological standards due to CSO.s. There are approximately 5,500 overflows that discharge to high-priority sites across England out of a total of around 15,000 CSO.s. Even further off, this must be achieved for all (100%) storm overflows discharging in or close to high-priority sites by 2045. WaSCs must achieve this target for all remaining storm overflow sites by 2050 [2].

From a public health perspective, the definition of "high-priority sites" is surely too restrictive, and, what about where people use the water for recreational purposes? Are the timescales too great? Under the plan, WaSCs must significantly reduce harmful pathogens from storm overflows discharging into and near designated bathing waters by either applying disinfection or reducing the frequency of discharges to meet Environment Agency standards by 2035. Again, this surely is not good enough.

Storm overflows will not be permitted to discharge above an average of ten rainfall events per year by 2050. With global heating and extreme weather, this will not require investment to future-proof the capacity of wastewater treatment works. The CSO.s were originally designed and intended to only operate in unusually heavy rainfall events, and evidence is that the CSO.s are currently operating in dry weather. This may also be in part a consequence of the sewerage infrastructure lacking the capacity to deal with the rate of flow from modern water usage. There must surely be some moves to improve the efficient use (reduction) of water too.

In addition to reducing the use of CSO.s under the plan, WaSCs will have to ensure all inland and coastal storm overflows have screening controls, but these will not only screen out pathogens, limiting the discharge of larger inorganic materials as well as faecal and organic solids.

The Government is required to review the targets in 2027, but as this is after the next General Election, it is to be hoped that this will be reviewed sooner.

Based on the modelled costs, it is anticipated that annual water bills averaged over the whole period to 2050 would eventually rise by £42 p.a. compared to current prices. There will be no bill impacts until 2025. The question arises, what about the polluter pays principle, and what about the profits and dividends that have been paid out since privatisation? Why should consumers be expected to pay for what is a public health measure that is required as a result of failures by the WaSCs and governments over the last decades?

Wet wipes contribute to around 93% of blockages in UK sewers and the creation of "fatbergs", according to Water UK. The government first said in 2018 that it planned to ban plastic from wet wipes and other products that get flushed down the toilet, and it announced this again in April 2023. In a 2021 consultation, 96% of people said they supported the idea, yet nothing happened. Earlier this year, the government decided against banning wet wipes following another consultation. In Wales, a ban has not yet been implemented, and the Scottish government consulted on a ban but has not taken further action.

Parliamentary Bills

There have also been recent attempts to improve legislative control over sewage pollution through amendments to the Environment Bill (but they were defeated by the Government, who introduced their own amendments), the Sewage (Inland Waters) Bill, which was introduced by the Duke of Wellington in the House of Lords in 2021 but has never progressed, and the Water Quality (Sewage Discharge) Bill.

The Labour Party tabled a motion in the House of Commons in April 2023 that sought to secure time to consider its Water Quality (Sewage Discharge) Bill that would require water companies to reduce discharges from storm overflows by 90% by the end of 2030 and impose automatic financial penalties for sewage dumping. However, MPs voted 290 to 188, a majority of 102, in favour of the Government's amendment to Labour's motion, which deleted mention of the Opposition's bid to introduce draft legislation; in effect, the Conservative Party rejected the move, with the Secretary of State saying the plan was "pointless because it is already being done", which, as you will see from the above, is not strictly true.

However, in a subsequent statement to Parliament, she referred to the plan discussed, which will require water companies to deliver an "infrastructure programme totalling an estimated £56 billion".

The Secretary of State announced that through the Environment Act 2021, the Government will legislate for "a clear target on storm overflow reduction in line with our Plan". This will also be backed by existing separate interim targets for bathing waters and our most precious habitats". This follows the introduction of monitoring in 2013, which will reach 100% by the end of 2023. It is also proposed to "reform penalties to make them easier to apply, including proposing an unlimited penalty" and "water companies provide action plans on every storm overflow by the summer".[4]

It would be a sign of commitment to improving water quality if the penalties for sewage pollution were substantially increased (currently limited to £250,000[5]), but there should also be the potential for custodial sentences.

The Government also has to encourage Ofwat to increase "materially the proportion of each company's capital investment devoted to improving water quality". The House of Commons Environmental Audit Committee has also called for the government to publish its assessment of "every possible option" to reduce pressures on the existing infrastructure while also assessing the case for "significant" capital work in its statutory plan to reduce storm overflow spills. As has been pointed out, the level of investment needed to deal with the worst CSO at £56 billion almost matches the £57 billion in dividends English WaSCs have paid to shareholders since privatisation.[6] Why does the government not put a cap on the payment of dividends until adequate controls on sewage discharges are in place?

Ofwat

Ofwat asked all companies to produce an action plan setting out how they would rapidly improve river health. As they finalise plans, they must demonstrate a commitment to public health that matches public expectations. They assess the water company business plans to ensure the targets are delivered and to "provide best value to customers and the environment, challenging companies to keep bill increases manageable for consumers".

Ofwat has been more concerned with water bills and economic regulation of the companies than their environmental performance. This led to the environmental campaign group Wild Justice seeking a judicial review of Ofwat's failure to monitor and take enforcement action against water firms that discharge raw sewage into waterways.

In 2021, the Environment Agency and Ofwat launched separate investigations into sewage treatment works. In November 2022, Ofwat's Chief Executive wrote to customers to provide an update of sorts [3]. When considering sewage discharges, it was accepted that this "causes more anger and questions". To help understand whether this is down to illegal activity with how companies manage their treatment, Ofwat has "made more than 30 evidence requests of companies and analysed over 3,000 pieces of evidence so far". This led to open enforcement cases against five companies: Anglian Water, Northumbrian Water, Thames Water, Wessex Water, and Yorkshire Water in March 2022. Although "these five companies were our initial focus, all wastewater companies remain part of our wider investigation". Continuing concern In June, growing concerns about environmental performance led Ofwat to open a further enforcement case against South West Water. At least it was recognised "that we (Ofwat) meet the high standards required for any enforcement action".

Ofwat is monitoring plans to improve river quality at no extra cost to customers and to reduce sewage discharges by 25% by 2025. There will be, from 2025, proposed compulsory annual targets for further improvement from 2025 (why not sooner?). Ofwat is now moving to make sure companies spend more of their shareholders' money to reduce the use of storm overflows with proposals to strengthen the ability "to take action against companies paying out excessive dividends while failing to deliver for customers and the environment". About time, one might say.

In May 2023, it was reported that UK water company dividends increased to £1.4 billion[7] in 2022, up from £540 million in 2021. These are higher than the headline dividends because of complex corporate structures with a number of subsidiaries, only one of which is regulated by Ofwat (the operating company). Dividends are paid internally and reduce the amount that can be invested. The "byzantine" structures are a concern to Ofwat as this means a lack of transparency, so it is said to be updating licence conditions so it can block dividends from 2025 if the company looks financially vulnerable and will also require boards to take account of environmental targets when making payments. Ofwat has said it does not recognise the distinction between internal (supposedly used to service debt, although there was no debt at privatisation) and external dividends and will take account of all dividends. Ofwat considers that companies have accumulated £60.6 billion in borrowing since privatisation, while total spending on wastewater infrastructure has "failed to rise significantly".

Environment regulators

The Environment Agency in England has had resources cut in recent years, and staffing in the environmental regulators is generally under pressure, but without effective and full enforcement of the provisions, there is less of an incentive for WaSCs and polluters to comply and direct sufficient investment to improving the sewerage infrastructure and preventing pollution.

In Wales, in ,2022 the Minister for Climate Change launched the Wales Better River Quality Taskforce. The taskforce brings together key players from the Welsh Government, Natural Resources Wales, Dŵr Cymru, Hafren Dyfrdwy, and Ofwat, with independent advice from Afonydd Cymru and the Consumer Council for Water. The taskforce has collaboratively developed action plans to gather greater evidence on the impact of CSO.s on rivers, reduce the impacts they cause, improve regulation, and educate the public on sewer misuse. A roadmap outlining these actions was published in July 2022[8] and a furtther report "was due" in March 2023.

In Scotland, in 2021, Scottish Environmental Protection Agency SEPA set out its expectations and timetable for a route map for Scottish Water to improve urban waters as part of the actions required in the River Basin Management Plan 2021–27.[9] This "highlighted the need for a step change in our efforts to tackle the most significant environmental impacts as soon as possible and to take a One Planet Prosperity approach to improve our urban waters for the long term".

SEPA appreciated that this was something that required concerted action and resources not only by Scottish Water but by others, including SEPA, the Scottish Government, Local Authorities, and customers. It was recognised that issues relevant to sewage discharges had emerged, such as microplastics, antimicrobial resistance, and an increase in wild swimming, which were not considered in the current legislation or in SEPA's current regulatory policy.

In December 2021, Scottish Water published a route map highlighting the need for investment actions required by it as a public body and responsible authority for River Basin Management Planning, as well as significant work needed with other partners to deliver long-term improvements.

In Northern Ireland Since April 2007, Northern Ireland Water Limited (NIW) has been responsible for regulating discharges from Wastewater Treatment Works. NIW is fully responsible for non-compliance and any pollution incidents caused by a failure to properly maintain and operate its water infrastructure. Both CSOs and Emergency Overflows (EOs) are part of Northern Ireland's sewerage system. Along with NIW, the Water Utility Regulation Group is assessing proposed upgrades to the sewerage systems of towns and cities across the region.

This is a long-term programme that addresses the impact of CSOs on complete sewerage systems and is guided by what is known as Urban Pollution Management methodology. Discharge standards for CSOs include minimum flows that the sewer must be capable of before spilling. For EOs, discharge standards relate to measures to be taken to ensure that there is no spillage following a breakdown.

On bathing waters affected by sewage pollution, the problem illustrated in *Anglian Water Service Ltd v Environment Agency* [2020] EWHC 3544 (Admin), [2021] All ER (D) 24 (Jan) where the regulations require the Agency to disregard samples taken when there has been exceptional weather even though there is a risk to public health, so that in the event the classification of the waters in question could not be downgraded. It seems that even when the Agency tries to provide important information to the public, the legislation is drafted so as to limit the extent to which public health is protected. Thus, perhaps the Bathing Water Regulations (and signage) need to be reviewed.

Local authorities

Local authorities in England and Wales, including county councils where they exist, have a part to play in ensuring that drains are maintained in good repair and do not leak, whether existing or new drainage. This also applies to Highway Drains that are the responsibility of the county councils.

Local authorities as well as environmental agencies need to make sure that septic tanks are working properly and are checked regularly. While new septic tanks are subject to building control (and unless a replacement) planning provisions, the Environment Agency may require the discharge to be connected to a sewer if it is reasonable to do so. There are also general, binding rules that govern the operation of existing septic tanks, depending on whether the discharge is to surface water or into the ground. If the general binding rules are met, there is no need for a permit; if not (or the septic tank deals with more than domestic sewage), then a permit is required from the Agency. In truth, it is more likely that the local authority, EHO (EHP), will know the location of septic tanks than the Agency.[10]

There is also a need for authorities at the district level to identify misconnections and use their powers as set out in Chapters 3 and 4 to have them remedied. It would make a lot of sense for these councils to work with the relevant environment agencies and the WaSCs on this. As has been pointed out, although the major culprits are the WaSCs when it comes to sewage discharges, EHOs can make a substantial contribution to raising awareness of the issue with the public by acting to identify and secure remedies where there are misconnections, especially when householders may be unaware that such a misconnection exists, and addressing exfiltration from drains (and as infiltration increases the flow and demands on treatment, it would help the WaSCs too).

As has been pointed out, surface water sewers that discharge to water courses were not transferred to the WaSCs, yet many householders will not be aware of where these sewers discharge. If these sewers only take surface water, that might not be a problem, but too often subsequent installations that require drainage can be connected, or polluting materials can be poured down surface water gullies on the misapprehension that the waste goes to treatment. As we have seen, the environmental agencies lack the resources to investigate and deal with pollution from these sources when there could be up to 500,000 such misconnections.

These sewers can also become blocked, which, in heavy rain, could cause flooding. There is, therefore, a need for local authorities, WaSCs, and environmental agencies to develop a joint strategy for identifying and securing remedial work. For local authorities, the powers in s.59 of the Building Act 1984 enable them to do so. Where there is a blockage in a private sewer, as illustrated in the *Swansea* case, the authority may serve notice only on those owners or occupiers of buildings served by the sewer up to the point where it is defective.

Local authorities have a public health responsibility, and while they may warn people where recreational waters (inland and coastal) are polluted by sewage, they also have a role to play in protecting both public health and local businesses where shellfish are harvested. The Food Standards Agency is directly responsible for decisions in relation to the classification and official control monitoring of shellfish and gives advice on the closure and re-opening of shellfish production and relay areas. Live bivalve molluscs include oysters (pacific and native), mussels, clams, cockles, and scallops. These are filter feeders and susceptible to picking up and accumulating toxins, chemical, or bacteriological contaminants from their environment.[11] These species can only be commercially harvested from classified production areas that are monitored. There are treatments that shellfish must undergo to reduce the level of microbiological contamination in them and ensure they are safe for placing on the market. Sampling for official controls is carried out by the local authority for the area where a shellfish bed is located. This is usually the EHO, and so they should be aware of any problems resulting from sewage pollution and work with other agencies to reduce sewage pollution.

As we have seen previously, local authorities are responsible for the signage at designated bathing waters, but that does not apply for other places where people may swim or undertake recreational activities on water. As a matter of public health, where anyone is likely to bathe or undertake recreational activities in or on the water, they should warn people of sewage pollution (the WasCs are unlikely to do so).

For these reasons, there is no reason why local councils, individually and collectively, should not be campaigning for improved sewage treatment. It is clear from this book that sewage pollution prejudices both public health and the amenity value of areas, including those where wild water swimming occurs, and that impacts local economies. This is why river pollution has become a leading issue on doorsteps in some areas during the countdown to the local elections in May 2023, and it is something that local councillors ought to take seriously in the future.

WASCs

In England, the companies have thus far moved very slowly to address the problems associated with the sewerage system. They seem to have only done the minimum required by the EA and Ofwat, as can be seen from the discussion above on dividends. Pressure is likely to increase, however, and action must go beyond monitoring all the CSOs.

Campaigners and NGOs

We have seen already, both in this book and in the media the importance of campaigning to get action from the government, environmental agencies, and companies themselves. Surfers Against Sewage is perhaps the best known of the campaign groups. They also provide useful information to the public on where there are polluted waters, and with the increased popularity of wild swimming, that is important.

While sewage pollution of our waters is important, we should not forget the other sources of water pollution that have led to the situation where, in England, only 758 out of 4,651 (16%) "water bodies" are of good or high ecological status and none are of good chemical status.[12,13] In Wales, it is suggested that 44.5% of rivers are in good ecological condition. In Scotland, 65.4% of our surface and groundwater water bodies are in good or better status.[14] In Northern Ireland, in 2018, 141 (31%) of river water bodies were classified as good or high.[15]

All this leaves a lot of scope for water campaigners to continue their work. They should be supported by local authorities, EHPs, their professional bodies, and all concerned with environmental and indeed public health.

The value of campaigning (including for water to gain Bathing Water status) can be gauged by the more than £1.6 billion that was announced in April 2023 to be invested by water companies in England in the next two years by the regulator, which is seen as a victory for campaigners pushing to clean up rivers. The investment by water companies has been brought forward to speed up projects to tackle pollution and drought. Residents in Ilkley, West Yorkshire, fought for their river to be the first in the UK to be given bathing water status,[16] and Yorkshire Water will now invest £67 million to cut sewage leaks from wastewater treatment plants. Ilkley Clean River Group said the plans were ambitious in their timescale, aiming for improvements to take shape in 2026.[17]

Matt Staniek of Windermere Lake Recovery has said Phosphorus is entering the catchment area in unsustainable quantities and destroying the fragile freshwater environment. He says "the problem of polluted waters has been caused by climate change, private sceptic tanks, and sewage being released into the lake, as in freshwater across the country, during storm overflows". High phosphorus levels in the water are feeding algae, stifling animal and vegetable organisms and biodiversity, and ultimately killing thousands of fish and freshwater species in the lake. He has used data from the EA in 2018 to illustrate that a phosphorus spike that was enough to drop the lake from 'good' to 'moderate' status on the Water Framework Directive.

As another example, Ashley Smith, the founder of the campaign group Windrush Against Sewage Pollution, has spent over six years investigating sewage pollution in the river. He argues that the public has been kept in the dark by the government and regulators. As he has pointed out, "Without bold and brutally honest media reporting, we would still be paddling around in ignorance and other people's sewage. Now we have to force the sewage scandal out as well with radical reform". One must agree with those views.

The public

It has been pointed out that part of the problem is down to the inadequate hydraulic capacity of the sewerage infrastructure, which leads to CSOs discharging in dry weather and causing properties to be affected by sewage flooding. There needs to be more emphasis on making people aware of what should not be put into the sewerage system (fats and grease, for example, that reduce sewer capacity further when they congeal), and ensuring all of us put wet wipes in waste bins or, better yet, that only rapidly biodegradable wet wipes are available would immediately assist in reducing avoidable outflow problems.

If the population was aware of the effects of flushing "non-flushable" products away and avoided their purchase, then manufacturers would soon stop making them. The government and companies, as well as campaigners, should be highlighting these issues and helping people reduce pressure on the sewerage infrastructure and the environment. While it is to be hoped that the Government does act on this, until it does, there will be increasing demands on sewers, sewerage, and the environment as it is, which will only be exacerbated further if we as individuals do not also take action.

Future pressures

What this book has shown is the problem with the existing and creaking infrastructure, which cannot cope as it is, but there will be increasing demands on the sewerage infrastructure, so if we are not to face a public health and environmental catastrophe, more has to be done and investment has to be increased. massively and regulation has to be greatly improved.

The population of the UK is currently increasing and is just over 67 million. In the past ten years, populations of all the nations have increased. The population of the UK is projected to increase by 3.2% in the first ten years of the projections, from an estimated 67.1 million in mid-2020 to 69.2 million in mid-2030.[18] This means that the demand for water will increase, as will the amount of sewage generated and passing into the sewerage system. This alone justifies increased investment in the sewerage infrastructure.

Then there is global heating, which in turn will lead to extreme weather and increased flooding events. Scientists at the Met Office Hadley Centre have shown evidence that days with extreme rainfall accumulations will become more frequent through the century [4]. The research used the record rainfall observed on 3 October 2020 as an example and found that while in a natural environment, with no influence from human-induced climate change, an event similar or more extreme would be a 1 in 300-year event, it is now a 1 in 100-year event in the current climate. By 2100, under a medium emissions scenario, that level of extreme daily rainfall could be seen every 30 years, making it ten times more likely than in a natural environment [4].

Perhaps we should be looking beyond reliance on a water-carrying sewerage system, expanding the use of SuDS as a matter of urgency, and looking at new ways of dealing with our waste products.

Even if the WaSCs were to be nationalised, we would need a massive programme of new work. The underinvestment goes back decades, and as has just been illustrated, demands on the sewerage infrastructure are only set to increase. Yet as George Monbiot has said,[19] as currently set up in England, "dividend incentives –profits versus public service – are lethal to the health of our rivers", one could add, and to public health too.

Notes

1 See https://www.theguardian.com/environment/2023/apr/04/therese-coffey-accused-of-throwing-in-the-towel-over-sewage-scandal

2 See: https://www.thetimes.co.uk/article/1cbd400a-d878-11ed-89ad-19e3cfc05db4?shareToken=9776454de947117f4f6f351292cde29c

3 See; Financial Times 21 April 2023 T https://www.ft.com/content/370854fc-a961-43c8-8cb1-79322c2b42cf

4 https://questions-statements.parliament.uk/written-statements/detail/2023-04-25/hcws735

5 It has been proposed by the government that there be unlimited fines and make "sure that money from higher fines and penalties - taken from water company profits, not customers - is channelled directly back into rivers, lakes and streams where it is needed" https://www.bbc.co.uk/news/science-environment-65145953.

6 https://www.theguardian.com/global/2022/sep/06/uk-government-defends-plan-to-reduce-sewage-discharges

7 Financial Times "UK water company dividends jump to £1.4bn despite criticism over sewage outflows" 8 May 2023.

8 https://naturalresourceswales.gov.uk/about-us/news-blog-and-statements/statements/wales-better-river-quality-taskforce/?lang=en

9 https://www.sepa.org.uk/environment/water/improving-urban-waters/

10 There are different provisions in different parts of the UK and registration, or consent may be required – see https://naturalresources.wales/permits-and-permissions/water-discharges-and-septic-tanks/register-your-septic-tank-or-small-sewage-treatment-plant/?lang=en; https://www.sepa.org.uk/regulations/water/septic-tanks-and-private-sewage-treatment-systems/, and https://www.daera-ni.gov.uk/articles/regulating-water-discharges. In England septic tanks needed to be upgraded by 2020. This did not apply in Scotland.

11 It is also a requirement to monitor classified production areas for marine biotoxins, phytoplankton and chemical contamination.

12 https://environment.data.gov.uk/catchment-planning/England/classifications

13 The Water Framework Directive classification scheme for water quality includes five status classes: 'high', 'good', 'moderate', 'poor' and 'bad'. 'High' status is defined as the biological, chemical and morphological conditions associated with no or very low human pressure (the reference condition). Assessment of quality is based on the amount of deviation from the reference condition; 'Good status' means 'slight' deviation, 'moderate status' means 'moderate' deviation etc.

14 https://www.sepa.org.uk/environment/water/aquatic-classification/

15 https://www.daera-ni.gov.uk/news/northern-ireland-water-framework-directive-statistics-report-2021-released

16 https://sites.google.com/view/cleanwharfeilkley/swimming-in-the-river

17 https://www.theguardian.com/environment/2023/apr/03/water-firms-invest-improvements-ofwat?ref=biztoc.com

18 https://www.ons.gov.uk/peoplepopulationandcommunity/populationandmigration/
populationprojections/bulletins/nationalpopulationprojections/2020basedinterim
19 Guardian 4 May 2023.

References

1 Giakournis T and Voulvoulis N, 2023, Combined sewer overflows: relating event
duration monitoring data to wastewater systems' capacity in England, *Environmental Science Water Research & Technology, Royal Society of Chemistry*, https://doi.
org/10.1039/d2ew00637e
2 Defra, 2022, *Storm Overflows Discharge Reduction Plan*, OGL, at https://assets.
publishing.service.gov.uk/government/uploads/system/uploads/attachment_data/
file/1101686/Storm_Overflows_Discharge_Reduction_Plan.pdf
3 Ofwat, 2022, *Water customers update on investigation into sewage treatment works*, at
https://www.ofwat.gov.uk/publication/water-customers-update-on-investigation-
into-sewage-treatment-works/
4 McCarthy M and Cotterill D et al., 2021, Record breaking daily rainfall in the
United Kingdon and the role of anthropogenic forcings, *Atmospheric Science Letter*, 22e1033. https://doi.org/10.1002/asl.1033

Index

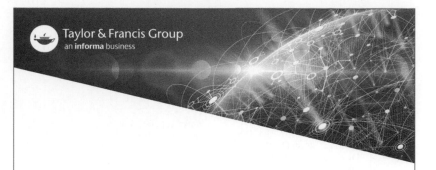